Bone Marrow Transplantation

AF880160

Under the educational grant of ASTA Medica AG

ASTA MEDICA
Ein Unternehmen der Degussa

U. W. Schaefer, D. W. Beelen

In collaboration with:
J. Neuser, H. Grosse-Wilde, H. Ottinger

Bone Marrow Transplantation

2nd, Revised Edition
17 illustrations, 3 in color, and 17 tables, 1996

KARGER

Basel · Freiburg · Paris · London · New York ·
New Delhi · Bangkok · Singapore · Tokyo · Sydney

Library of Congress Cataloging-in-Publication Data

Schaefer, U. W. (Ulrich W.)
[Knochenmarktransplantation. English]
Bone marrow transplantation / U. W. Schaefer, D. W. Beelen; in collaboration with
Jürgen Neuser, Hans Grosse-Wilde, Helmut Ottinger. -- 2nd rev. ed.
X+126 p. 13,5 × 19,5 cm.
ISBN 3-8055-6308-6 (softcover)
1. Bone marrow -- Transplantation. I. Beelen, D. W. (Dietrich W.). II. Neuser, Jürgen.
III. Grosse-Wilde, Hans. IV. Ottinger, Helmut. V. Title.
[DNLM: 1. Bone Marrow Transplantation. WH 380 S294b 1996a]
RD 123.5.S3313 1996
617.4'4 -- dc20
DNLM/DLC for Library of Congress 96-20422 CIP

Drug Dosage. The authors and the publisher have exerted every effort to ensure that drug selection and dosage set forth in this text are in accord with current recommendations and practice at the time of publication. However, in view of ongoing research, changes in government regulations, and the constant flow of information relating to drug therapy and drug reactions, the reader is urged to check the package insert for each drug for any change in indications and dosage and for added warnings and precautions. This is particularly important when the recommended agent is a new and/or infrequently employed drug.

Printed in Germany by Konkordia Druck GmbH, D–77815 Bühl
ISBN 3–8050–6308–6

Contents

Preface to the 2nd Edition

This booklet is aimed to provide a short introduction to the rapidly developing field of allogeneic and autologous bone marrow or peripheral blood progenitor cell transplantation. It is especially dedicated to those readers who are not immediately involved in the treatment of and the care for transplant patients. The authors were therefore endeavored to restrict the information to the most important basic principles, clinical issues, and future developments. For those readers who would like to get a deeper or more scientific insight into the transplantation of hematopoietic cells, the comprehensive textbooks mentioned at the end of this booklet are strongly recommended.

The authors sincerely hope that the 2nd edition of this booklet will contribute to the understanding of essential aspects of the biology of hematopoietic cell transplantation and of the clinical management of transplant patients.

November 1995

Ulrich W. Schaefer
Dietrich W. Beelen

Department of Bone Marrow Transplantation
University Hospital of Essen
Germany

1. Introduction

1.1. Background

The story of bone marrow transplantation began only a few decades ago. Around the turn of the century, doctors began trying to treat blood diseases with orally administered raw or cooked animal spleen. The first attempt to treat aplastic anemia with intravenous injections of bone marrow cells from a person of the same blood group was published in 1939.

Serious animal experiments, however, were only begun in the 1950s by Jacobson and Lorenz. These experiments showed that death could be prevented in rodents that had received total-body irradiation (TBI) if they were given intravenous spleen or bone marrow cells from syngeneic donors. For quite some time there was a lively controversy whether this protection was the result of hormones or of the intravenous cells themselves.

Lorenz favored hormonal factors. Cole, and later Alpen and Baum, supported the cell-replacement theory, which later received additional support from similar experiments in mice and dogs.

Even during these early experiments it was noted that, although genetically identical spleen or bone marrow cells definitely protected the animals from death after irradiation, animals which had received genetically different cell material and had shown a temporary improvement, subsequently died nonetheless. In the years that followed, many authors examined and described a remarkable biologic phenomenon: after TBI, the destroyed hematopoiesis could be replaced by infusion of a few blood-generating precursor cells from bone marrow or spleen. In 1956, Ford introduced the expression "radiation chimaera", to characterize the situation in which the hematopoiesis of an irradiated animal has been completely replaced through injections of marrow from another animal. The name has its origin in Greek mythology where the chimaera was a being made up of body parts from a lion, a goat, and a serpent. In medicine, the term "chimaeras" describes the coexistence of cell populations from different individuals within a single organism. In nature, a hematopoietic chimaerism sometimes occurs in heterozygous twins when fetal vessel anastomoses result in an exchange of individual blood-building cells.

Normally, genetically different individuals are not immunologically tolerant to each other. In bone marrow transplantation, a hematopoietic chimaerism can only be achieved after an intense immunosuppressive treatment, such as TBI. The animal experiments of the 1950s showed that the use of genetically different bone marrow could not prevent death after TBI in each case. Often, in spite of hematopoietic restitution, a secondary disease developed that was called "secondary disease", "runt disease" or "wasting disease". The very thorough animal experiments conducted by van Bekkum and his work group in Rijswijk (The Netherlands) contributed significantly to our understanding of the complex biological reactions following TBI and bone marrow transplantation. A distinction was made between primary radiation-induced damage and the immunological side effects of bone marrow transplantation. Today, two distinct immune reactions are recognized: Host-versus-graft reaction (HvGR) and graft-versus-host reaction (GvHR). Secondary disease after transplantation of hematopoietic cells in a recipient pretreated with TBI is the result of a GvHR in which the immune cells in the graft react aggressively to the recipient organism. This type of immune defense reaction is to be expected when the donor and recipient are genetically different. When donor and recipient belong to the same species, bone marrow transplantation is called allogeneic transplantation. In case of transplantation between different species it is called xenogeneic transplantation. If the donor and recipient are one and the same individual, it is called autologous transplantation. In genetically identical individuals, for example identical twins, it is called syngeneic, or isologous transplantation. After autologous or syngeneic transplantations, immune-defense reactions do not occur.

1.2. First Clinical Trials

After work on animals had provided an experimental basis, the knowledge obtained therefrom was applied to the treatment of humans with life-threatening hematologic disorders. The impetus was provided by a nuclear reactor accident in Yugoslavia. Six people who had been exposed to radiation were flown to Paris and treated by a team of French and Yugoslav doctors led by Jammet and Mathé. Five patients received bone marrow transplantations from blood-group-identical donors. Four patients survived and 1 patient died. There was some evidence of a temporary graft function in surviving patients. In the final analysis, however, the value of bone marrow transplantation continued to remain unclear.

In 1970, Bortin published a survey of 203 bone marrow transplantations carried out between 1950 and 1962. The results were not encouraging. Of 203 patients, 152 had died by the time of the case study concerned. In at least 125 patients, engraftment was not achieved. Chimaerism was identified in only 11 cases, and only 3 patients were still alive when Bortin's survey was published.

Until the end of the 1960s, bone marrow transplantation received little attention. In the 1970s the significance of histocompatibility testing was recognized, and the modern era of bone marrow transplantation began. In the selection of donors, preference was given to family members whose peripheral blood cells showed the same reaction patterns as the patient's own complement-dependent lymphocytotoxicity assay (antigens recognized by cytotoxic antibodies). The first successful bone marrow transplantation was reported by Robert Good's group and involved a child with severe combined immunodeficiency. In this case, a sibling donor was chosen on the basis of the antigen pattern of the major histocompatibility complex, known as the HLA system.

Results continued to improve in the 1970s, due mainly to refined methods for histocompatibility testing, advances in the supportive therapy of aplastic syndromes through transfusions of thrombocytes and granulocyte concentrates, and decontamination and isolation in germ-free rooms.

In the last 10 years, improvements have continued, including moving up the time of transplantation to the early phase of disease, introduction of fractionated TBI, and the use of the immunosuppressive agent ciclosporin. Bone marrow transplantation has now acquired a standard place in the treatment of severe aplastic anemia, severe combined immunodeficiency syndromes, acute leukemia and chronic myeloid leukemia (CML). At the end of 1990, about 40,000 bone marrow transplantations had been performed worldwide. At present, a yearly rate of about 5,000 transplantations is expected. Since new indications continue to be found and transplantations using the patients' own marrow (autologous marrow transplantation), as well as transplantations with marrow from unrelated donors, are being performed with increasing frequency, an increase in the importance of this form of therapy can be anticipated.

The first bone marrow transplantation was performed by our group in Essen in 1975. In the years which followed, the project was systematically expanded and at present about 120 allogeneic transplantations are being performed per year. The largest and most experienced center in the world is the Fred Hutchinson Cancer Research Center in Seattle, WA.

2. Immunological Aspects of Bone Marrow Transplantation

H. Ottinger, H. Grosse-Wilde

This chapter will introduce readers to the immunological phenomena associated with the transplantation of allogeneic bone marrow.

2.1. There Are Basic Differences between Transplantation of Bone Marrow and of Solid Organs

The major immunological differences between the transplantation of solid organs (kidney, liver, etc.) and allogeneic bone marrow transplantation (BMT) have been recently summarized by Paul Martin (FHCRC, Seattle, WA) as follows:

In case of a solid-organ transplantation the graft contains only a small number of cells with immunological competence, and the immune system remains of recipient origin. Consequently, after transplantation of solid organs the immune reactions are predominantly operating in host-versus-graft (HvG) direction and may result in graft rejection. To prevent this major complication of a solid-organ transplantation, a lifelong administration of immunosuppressive medication is necessary.

In case of allogeneic BMT, however, the graft contains high numbers of immunocompetent cells. Thus, prior to BMT, the immune system of the host (if functioning) has to be eliminated (and not only suppressed !) by a preparative therapy called "conditioning". After a temporary state of severe immunodeficiency, immunological functions will be gradually reconstructed in the recipient, but notably by immunocompetent cells of donor origin (immune reconstitution). Since some immunocompetent cells of recipient origin survive the conditioning, immune reactions in HvG direction are also possible after BMT and may cause graft rejection. However, due to conditioning, these reactions are mainly operative in graft-versus-host (GvH) direction post BMT. This GvH reaction may cause specific lesions in the recipient, collectively named graft-versus-host disease (GvHD), but it may also exert a protective effect against relapse in patients transplanted for malignancies, called graft-versus-leukemia (GvL) effect. After BMT, immunosuppressive therapy is also necessary. In contrast to solid-organ transplantation, however, it is primarily administered to prevent GvHD and can be finally discontinued in virtually all patients, since post-BMT it is only a question of time until a state of immunological tolerance is achieved between the marrow donor and the recipient.

2.2. Major and Minor Histocompatibility Antigens Play a Crucial Role for the Outcome of Allogeneic BMT

A major cause of lethal complications after BMT are immune reactions causing GvHD or graft rejection. These complications occur if the donor and the recipient are not sufficiently matched for their "histocompatibility". Thus, we start our discussion on immunological phenomena associated with BMT by a short review on histocompatibility (transplantation) antigens. Antigenic differences among members of the same species are called alloantigens. Histocompatibility antigens are (traditionally) defined as those alloantigens on a graft that are responsible for graft rejection (graft failure mediated by the immune system of the host). In context of BMT, this definition is extended to alloantigens inducing either graft rejection or GvHD or the GvL effect. For genetical and functional reasons the histocompatibility antigens are grouped into "major" and "minor" antigens.

2.2.1. Major Histocompatibility Antigens in Humans Are the HLA Class I and II Molecules

The major histocompatibility antigens are a group of highly polymorphic glycoproteins exerting defined biological functions: They harbor peptides derived from self or foreign protein antigens, bring them up to the cell surface and present them to immunocompetent T cells. Due to this, they play a central role in the physiology of the immune system and are the major barrier for transplantation.

The genetics of HLA molecules are well established. All genes encoding for major histocompatibility antigens are located within a small section of a single chromosome, called the major histocompatibility complex (MHC). In humans, the MHC is named HLA (human leukocyte antigens). The HLA complex is located on the short arm of chromosome 6. It encompasses about 4,000 kilobase pairs (kBp), which is about 0.1% of the total human genome, and can be subdivided into the class I, class II and class III regions as shown in figure 1.

The telomeric class I region consists of approximately 1,900 kBp of DNA and contains beside other genes and non-expressed pseudogenes three well-characterized HLA gene loci, designated as A, B and C. These loci encode for the α or heavy chain of the HLA-A, HLA-B and HLA-C antigens, respectively. Each α-chain molecule has to assemble with a β- or light chain to form a complete HLA antigen molecule. The β-chain of HLA class I antigens, also known as β_2-microglobulin, is not encoded in the HLA complex but on chromosome 15. It is established in clinical studies that HLA-A and HLA-B antigens are relevant for the outcome of BMT, whereas the role of HLA-C molecules remains to be determined.

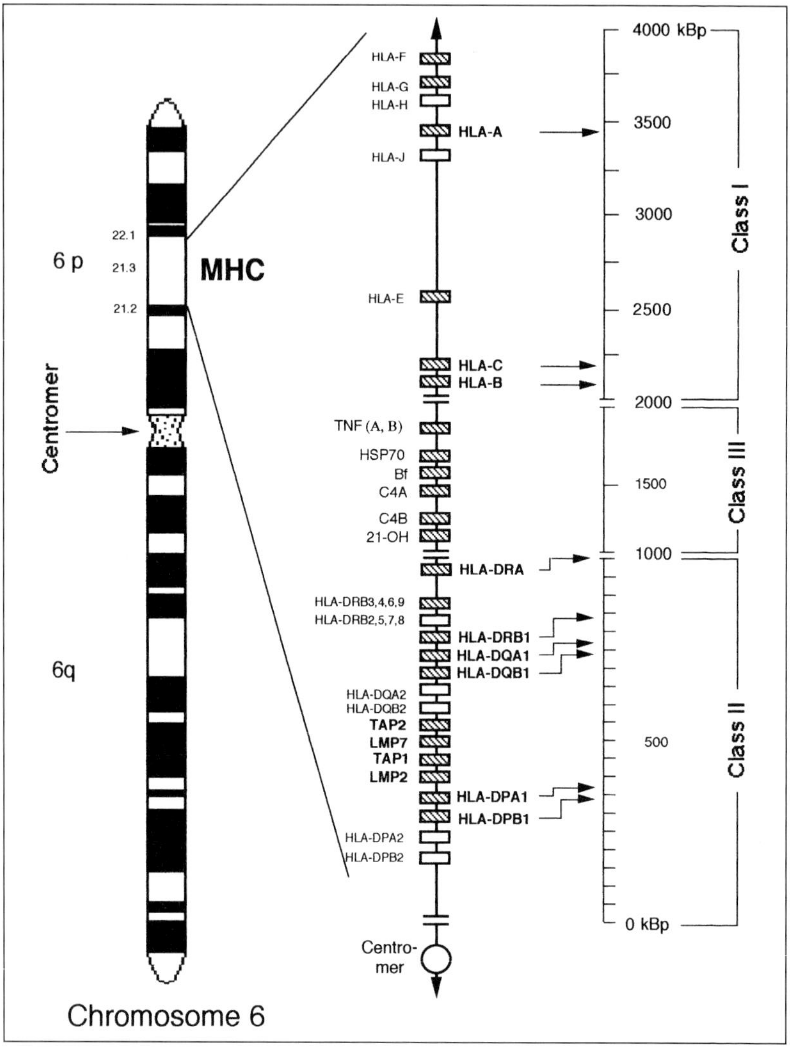

Fig. 1. Organization of the major histocompatibility complex (MHC) in humans. The human MHC (HLA-Complex) is located on the short arm of chromosome 6 (6p). The HLA-A, -B, -C and HLA-DRA1, -DRB1, -DQA1, -DQB1, and -DPA1, -DPB1 genes encode for the HLA-A, -B, -C and HLA-DR, -DQ, -DP antigens, respectively. The products of class II TAP1, 2 and LMP1, 7 genes are involved in antigen processing, whereas class III genes do not encode für HLA or HLA-related molecules. For details see text. Genes = ▨; pseudogenes (not expressed) = ▭.

The more centromeric class II region spans about 1,000 kBp of DNA and contains beside other genes, mentioned below, the α-chain and the β-chain genes of the HLA-DR, HLA-DQ, and HLA-DP antigens. The organization of the HLA-DR gene cluster is complex: One α-chain gene (DRA) and 9 different β-chain genes (DRB1, DRB3, DRB4, DRB6, DRB9; pseudogenes: DRB2, DRB5, DRB7, DRB8) have been identified. The number of existing β- chain genes varies from one individual to another (range: 2–5). It applies to the particular DRB1 allele being present, which other β-chain loci coexist with the DRB1 locus. The DRA,DRB1-encoded molecules are the classic serological HLA-DR specificities, whereas the DRA,DRB3-, DRA,DRB4- and DRA,DRB5-encoded HLA-DR molecules are known as the HLA-DR52, HLA-DR53 and HLA-DR51 specificities, respectively. For HLA-DQ and HLA-DP one α- and one β-chain gene (DQA1, DQB1; DPA1, DPB1) as well as one α- and one β-chain pseudogene (DQA2, DQB2; DPA2, DPB2) are identified. Whereas the HLA-DR and HLA-DQ antigens have a major impact on the success of BMT, HLA-DP molecules are obviously of minor importance.

The class III region is located between the class I and class II regions, stretches over approximately 680 kBp of DNA, and contains about 40 genes. These genes do not code for histocompatibility antigens, but for components of the complement system (C4, C2 and Bf), tumor necrosis factor (TNF) α and β, and other proteins.

HLA class I and class II molecules present peptides derived from antigens to T cells, but differ in structure, tissue distribution and function. HLA class I as well as class II antigens are heterodimeric glycoproteins (molecules composed of two different, noncovalently bound α- and β-chains) that are displayed on the cell surface in order to present peptides derived from antigens to T cells. Nevertheless, the two classes of HLA molecules differ with regard to (i) molecular structure, (ii) tissue distribution, and (iii) biological function. The molecular structures of class I and class II molecules are shown in figure 2. While class I molecules are distributed on virtually all nucleated cells and platelets, the expression of class II molecules is confined to cells with special immunological functions such as B cells, activated T cells, monocytes, macrophages, Langerhans cells in the skin and interdigitating dendritic cells in the lymph nodes. As detailed below, the main biological function of HLA class I molecules is the presentation of peptides derived from endogenous (intracellular) antigens to the CD8+ subset of T cells, whereas class II molecules present peptides derived from exogenous antigens to CD4+ T cells.

Presentation of antigen-derived peptides by HLA to T cells requires "antigen processing". Antibodies can directly detect target epitopes on intact antigens in the absence of HLA molecules. T cells, however, can recognize their antigens only in association with HLA molecules, a phenomenon called "MHC restriction of T-cell recognition", and the T-cell response is best, if "non-self" peptides are bound to "self"

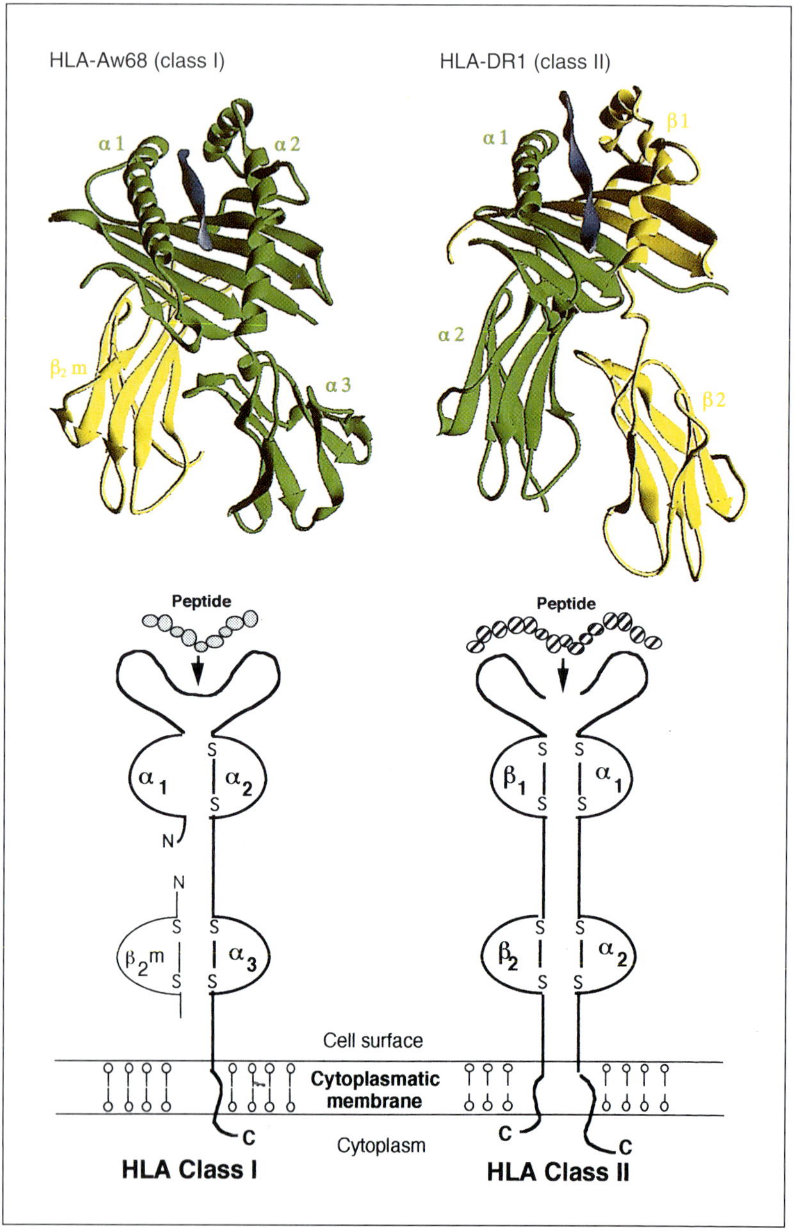
HLA-Aw68 (class I)
HLA-DR1 (class II)
α 1
α 2
β_2 m
α 3
β1
α 1
α 2
β2
Peptide
Peptide
α_1
α_2
N
N
β_2m
α_3
β_1
α_1
β_2
α_2
Cell surface
Cytoplasmatic membrane
Cytoplasm
C
C
C
HLA Class I
HLA Class II

HLA molecules. Since intact proteins are "too large" to complex with HLA molecules, they have to be "processed". This means that antigens of (glyco)protein nature undergo enzymatic cleavage, and selected antigen-derived peptides are subsequently intercalated into HLA molecules in order to be inspected by T cells through their respective T-cell receptors.

Processed endogenous antigens are preferentially presented by HLA class I molecules to CD8+ T cells. Endogenous antigens (proteins synthesized by the cell) are cleaved into peptides within the cytoplasma by a proteolytic complex, called the proteasome (figure 3). It is composed of subunits, named low-molecular mass polypeptides (LMP). The generated peptides are transported from the cytoplasm into the lumen of the endoplasmatic reticulum (ER) by means of an ATP-dependent membrane-spanning complex, named transporters associated with antigen processing (TAP). Within the ER, the peptides assemble with newly synthesized class I α- and β-chains to form complete and stable HLA class I molecules. Finally, peptide-loaded class I molecules are brought up to the cell surface by still unknown mechanisms. Three details of this process deserve being mentioned: (i) the presence of peptides is required for the stable assembling of class I molecules and their transport to the cell surface, (ii) HLA class I molecules bind peptides of 8–11 residues in length, and (iii) there are "allele-specific binding motifs", i.e., the amino acid sequence of the class I α-chain (which is unique for each HLA antigen) dictates, through crucial "anchor" and "co-anchor" positions, which group of peptides can intercalate. Obviously, LMP and TAP play a role in the generation of "correct" peptides and their transport into the ER. Interestingly, their encoding genes (TAP1, TAP2; LMP2, LMP7) are mapped within the MHC class II region (fig. 1).

Processed exogenous antigens are preferentially presented by HLA class II molecules to CD4+ T cells. Exogenous antigens (circulating proteins), taken up into the cell by pinocytosis or phagocytosis, are found to be incorporated within endosomes and phagosomes, as shown in figure 4. Within these cellular compartments the pro-

Fig. 2. The molecular structure of HLA class I and HLA class II antigens. Ribbon diagrams as determined by X-ray crystallography (top) and schematic views (bottom) of a class I (left) and a class II (right) molecule. The transmembrane and intracytoplasmatic domains are not visualized in the crystal structures. The class I α-chain has three globular domains (α_{1-3}) and is associated with the non-MHC-encoded β_2-microglobulin (β_2m). The class II α-chain and the shorter class II β-chain both have two globular domains termed $\alpha_{1,2}$ and $\beta_{1,2}$, respectively. Intra-chain disulfide bonds are indicated as -S–S-. The peptide binding groove consists of a β-pleated sheet on the bottom, and the α_1, and α_2 helices (in case of class I) and the α_1 and β_2 helices (in case of class II) on the sides. Ribbon diagrams are reprinted from Stern LJ, Wiley DC: Antigenic peptide binding by class I and class II histocompatibility proteins. Structure 1994; 2: 245–251, with kind permission from Current Biology Ltd., London.

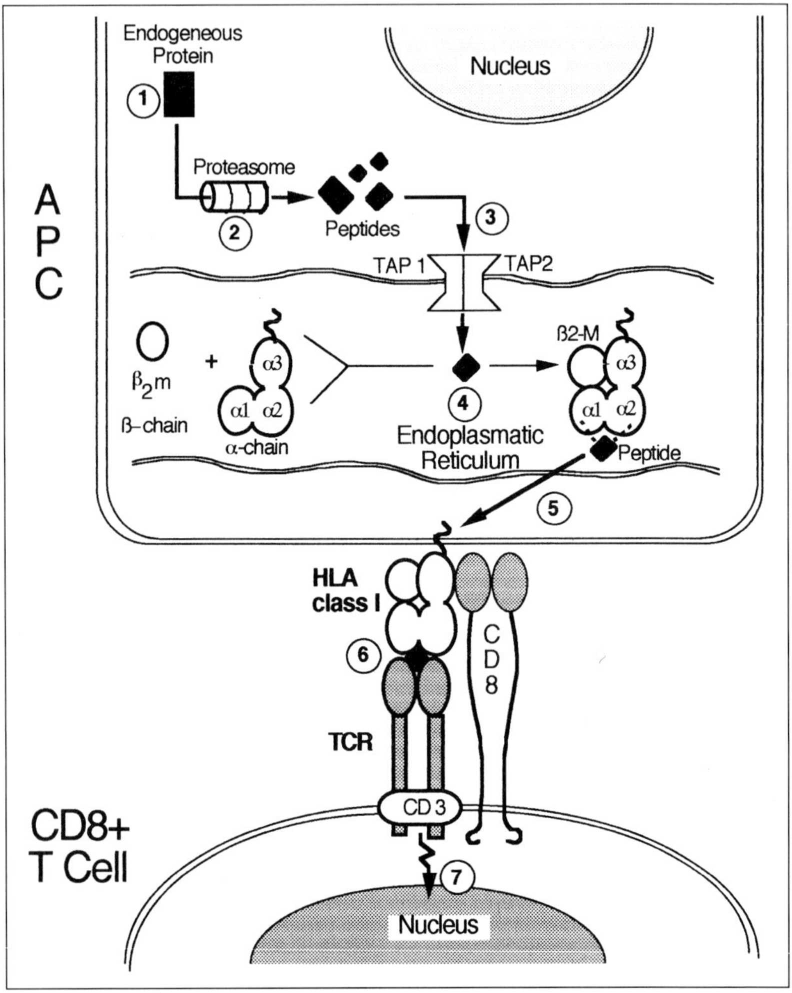

Fig. 3. Processing of an endogenous protein within an antigen-presenting cell (APC) and presentation of an antigen-derived peptide by HLA class I of the APC to a CD8+ T cell. Cleavage of an APC-derived protein antigen (1) by the cytoplasmatic proteasome complex (2). Translocation of an antigen-derived peptide into the endoplasmatic reticulum (ER) by means of TAP 1, 2 peptide transporter molecules (3). Formation of a peptide/HLA class I (α-chain, β-chain) complex (4). Arrival of this complex at the APC surface (5). Recognition of this complex by a CD8+ T cell (6), i.e., signal 1 for T-cell activation (7). TCR = T-cell receptor; CD8 and CD3 = TCR-associated proteins.

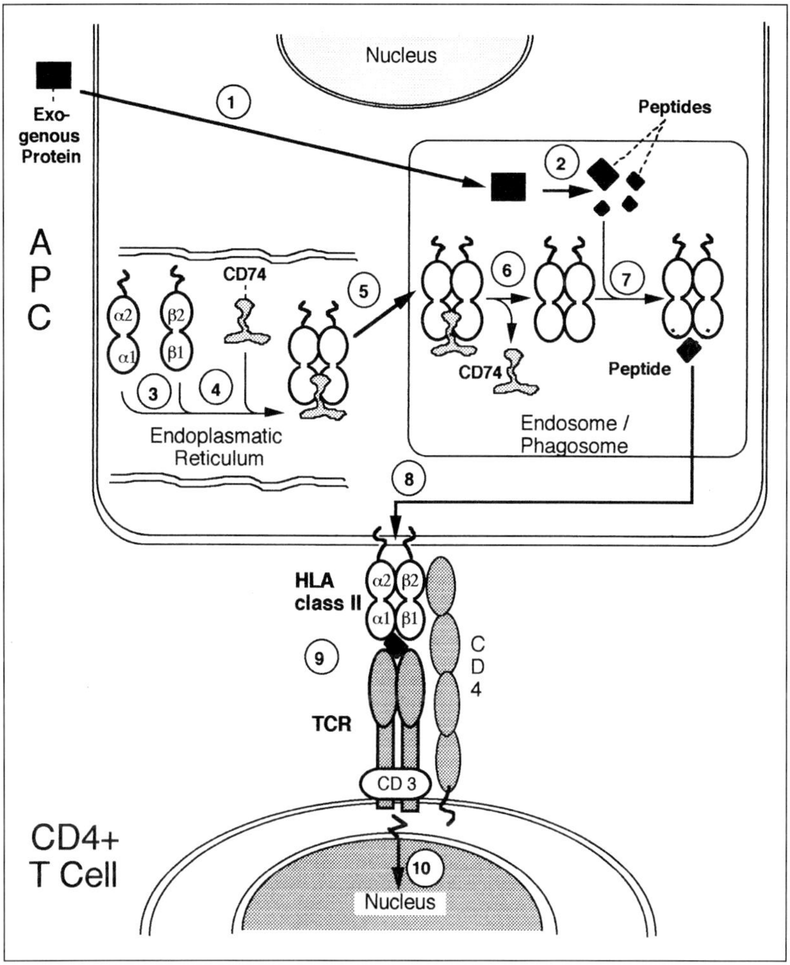

Fig. 4. Processing of an exogenous protein by an antigen-presenting cell (APC) and presentation of an antigen-derived peptide by HLA class II of the APC to a CD4+ T cell. Encorporation of a circulating antigen into the endosome/phagosome compartment of the APC (1), where degradation into peptides occurs (2). Association of class II HLA α- and β-chains (3) and the invariant chain (CD74) in the endoplasmatic reticulum (4). Translocation of the resulting trimolecular complex into the phagosome/endosome compartment (5), where CD74 is removed (6). Formation of an antigen-derived peptide/HLA class II molecule complex (7). Arrival of this complex at the cell surface (8), and recognition of this complex by CD4+ T cells (9), i.e., signal 1 for T-cell activation (10). TCR = T-cell receptor; CD3 and CD4 = TCR-associated proteins.

teins are enzymatically cleaved. The resulting peptides wait to be loaded into class II molecules which are derived from the ER. As for class I molecules, the assembly of newly synthesized class II α- and β-chains to intact class II molecules occurs within the ER but, in contrast to class I molecules, independently of the presence of peptides. After assembly the class II molecules immediately combine with a monomorphic glycoprotein, named the HLA class II γ- or invariant chain (CD74), which is encoded on chromosome 5. CD74 prevents binding of peptides to class II molecules within the ER. The resulting trimolecular complex (α+β+CD74) is then transported from the ER via the Golgi and Transgolgi networks into the endosomes and lysosomes. Here, class II molecules are allowed to bind to their peptides after proteolytic removal of CD74. Finally, peptide-loaded class II molecules are translocated to the cell surface. Peptides bound to class II molecules are generally longer than 9 amino acids and, in contrast to HLA class I associated peptides, are more heterogeneous in size (10–35 amino acid residues). Position-specific anchor residues and allele-specific binding motives have also been identified for class II - peptide interactions. Thus, if one and the same (exogenous or endogenous) antigen is processed by HLA-different individuals, different peptides (intercalated in different HLA molecules) may be presented to the T-cell receptor repertoires of these individuals.

T cells recognizing an HLA/peptide molecule complex may respond in different ways. If the T-cell receptor of a CD4+ or CD8+ T cell binds to an appropriate HLA molecule/peptide complex on the surface of an antigen-presenting cell (APC), the T cell will "respond". The quality of the response, however, may differ considerably and is dependent on the developmental and functional state of the T cell and the type of APC being involved. Under which conditions one and the same HLA molecule/peptide complex may contribute to T-cell activation, T-cell triggering (execution of an effector cell function) or T-cell tolerance will be discussed in paragraph 2.3.

To conclude our review on HLA molecules, we focus on the "polymorphism" and the way in which HLA antigens are inherited. Both topics are essential for the strategy of marrow donor search, which will be discussed in chapter 3. It is well established that one and the same gene may occur in two or more different forms, i.e., may code for different gene products (phenotypes). If the resulting different phenotypes are observed in the population in frequencies that cannot be explained solely by the rare event of gene mutation, the respective gene is called polymorphic and the corresponding different variants of the gene are called alleles.

Different alleles are defined by different sequences of nucleotides within the coding regions of the gene. The most polymorphic system in the human genome with hundreds of alleles is the HLA region. The listing of currently (March 1994) recognized HLA class I and class II alleles (WHO Nomenclature Committee for Factors of the HLA System) includes a total number of 406 expressed alleles (A: 50, B: 97, C: 34, DRA: 2, DRB1: 106, DRB3: 4, DRB4: 5, DRB5: 5, DRB6: 3, DRB7: 2, DQA1:

15, DQB1: 26, DPA1: 8, and DPB1: 44 alleles). Each HLA allele is designated by the encoding gene locus and an individual combination of 4 arabic numbers preceded by an asterix, e.g., HLA-A*0101, HLA-DRB1*1501, etc. Fortunately, not all of the recognized HLA alleles are clinically relevant since some of them encode for silent substitutions (tables 1 and 2 of chapter 3). Most of the HLA alleles occur in all ethnic groups, but the frequencies of a given allele may vary considerably between Caucasians, Orientals, Blacks, Native Americans, Asians and Hispanics. This fact is of importance for unrelated bone marrow donor search, since the vast majority of volunteers provided by the donor registries are Caucasians.

The diploid genes encoding for HLA class I and class II antigens are codominantly expressed on the cell surface. Thus, one paternal and one maternal set of HLA-A, -B, -C, -DR, -DQ, and -DP molecules are displayed on the cell surfaces. The combination of these two sets of HLA molecules is called the HLA phenotype of an individual.

The HLA class I and class II alleles, and in between the class III alleles, are normally inherited as a unit ("en bloc") making up an HLA haplotype. Each individual inherits one (out of two) HLA haplotype(s) from his/her mother and one (out of two) HLA haplotype(s) from his/her father (see fig. 6), making up the HLA genotype of an individual. The chance that two siblings are genotypically HLA-identical is thus 1:4 (Mendelian inheritance). Recombination of genetic material between homologous chromosomes during meiotic cell division is called "crossing over". Crossing-over events between HLA genes do occur, but their incidence is rare (approximately 2% between HLA-A and HLA-DQ). The HLA haplotype frequencies found in a population can be higher or lower than one would expect on the basis of the observed HLA allele frequencies. This phenomenon of preferred combinations of certain alleles within an HLA haplotype is called linkage disequilibrium or non-random gametic association, and substantially influences extended family and unrelated bone marrow donor search. The two most common Caucasian haplotypes are HLA-A1,B8,DR3,DQ2 and HLA-A3,B7,DR2, DQ1.

2.2.2. Minor Histocompatibility Antigens (Non-HLA Antigens) May Be Neither Weak Nor Minor

Clinical data show that graft rejection or GvHD may also occur in BMT from genotypically or phenotypically HLA-identical donors, but not in monozygotic twins. This observation points to the existence of antigens with histocompatibility function encoded outside the HLA complex. These non-HLA histocompatibility antigens are collectively named "minor histocompatibility antigens" (mH). With two exceptions, namely the antigens encoded by the y chromosome (H-Y) and the human monocyte alloantigens (HMA), the genetics and molecular structure of mH are unknown in humans. In mice, more than 40 not genetically linked loci have been identified to encode for mH, and some mH have been identified to be endogenous peptides (including peptides of retroviral origin) presented to T cells by MHC molecules. Cumulative mH differences can lead to graft rejection or GvHD to an extent seen in HLA-mismatched transplants. Since no reliable method is established in humans to detect donor vs. recipient mH differences prior to transplantation, the mH are a dark side of the current clinical histocompatibility testing.

2.3. Alloreactivity is a Basic Capacity of the Immune System, and Graft Rejection, GvHD and GvL Are Special Manifestations of Alloreactivity

Immune reactivity denotes the capacity of the immune system to react against non-self (alloreactivity) and self antigens in case of autoreactivity. The cellular basis of alloreactivity is the same, irrespective of whether the immune system reacts against infectious agents like bacteria, viruses, and fungi, or, in case of allogeneic BMT, against mismatched histocompatibility antigens exhibited by the graft, the host or the tumor. Thus, before discussing the immunological details of allograft rejection, GvHD, and GvL, we like to outline the general principles of alloreactivity.

T cells play the central role in alloreactivity. Alloreactivity is mediated by T cells, B cells and natural killer (NK) cells. Since T cells play the central role, we start with the definition of the different subtypes of T cells. Lymphoid progenitors destined to become T cells are derived from bone marrow stem cells and migrate to the thymus. Thymocytes are immature T cells developing in the thymus. While most thymocytes are deleted, only 3% (1 million/day in young mice) are selected for export to the peripheral blood and lymphatic tissues (paragraph 2.8). Mature peripheral T cells may be either "virgin" or "experienced". While a virgin (naive) T cell has not yet encountered its antigen peptide, experienced T cells have responded at least once. Mature (virgin or experienced) T cells may exist either in a resting ("precursor cell") state or in an activated ("effector cell") state. In contrast to resting experienced T cells ("memory cells"), effector T cells are short-lived. They may either fulfil their biological function (i.e., lysis of target cells, release of cytokines, etc.) and die, or they have to return into the resting state. Mature T cells (irrespective of whether virgin or experienced) are either positive for the CD4 or CD8 antigen. CD4 and CD8 are T-cell-receptor-associated adhesion molecules ("co-receptors") that bind to monomorphic regions of HLA class II and class I molecules, respectively. Consequently, CD8+ T cells will recognize antigen-derived peptides in association with HLA class I molecules, whereas CD4+ T cells will detect peptides bound to HLA class II molecules.

Activation of T cells requires two signals. The T-cell response to an antigen challenge includes activation and clonal proliferation of "precursor" cells and their differentiation into antigen-specific effector cells. Activation of T cells requires two signals, namely binding of the T-cell receptor to the appropriate HLA/peptide antigen complex (signal 1) and costimulation (signal 2) offered by the antigen-presenting cell (APC). Costimulatory signals are provided by various surface molecules on APCs (e.g., CD 80 or CD 86, also known as B7-1 and B7-2) interacting with their cognate ligands on T cells (e.g. CD 28). Virgin and experienced T cells have different requirements of costimulation: Virgin T cells accept signal 2 only from "professional" APC (interdigitating dendritic cells residing in the T-cell-dependent areas of lymphatic tissues and possibly also macrophages); in contrast, experienced T cells accept signal 2 from professional as well as non-professional APCs (B cells, monocytes, etc.). Notably, recognition of signal 1 in the absence of signal 2 leads to a long-lived state of antigen-specific T-cell hyporesponsiveness. We will come back to these points when discussing GvHD (paragraph 2.5) and tolerance after BMT (paragraph 2.8).

Activated T cells proliferate and differentiate into effector T cells in response to cytokines. Whereas resting T cells are confined to the recirculating lymphocyte pool (blood, lymphoid tissues, and lymph fluids), activated T cells have the capacity to cross capillary borders and to disseminate throughout the body with a notable tendency to finally home to the gut, skin, liver, and lung. Activation of T cells results in a state of cellular responsiveness to exogenous or endogenous cytokines, such as IL-2 and IL-12, which promote proliferation and differentiation. Once being activated and differentiated, effector T cells fulfil their biological functions in the absence of further costimulation if triggered by signal 1.

Activated T cells may differentiate into different types of effector cells. There are cytotoxic T lymphocytes (CTL) which are able to kill their target cells directly (generation of perforin and granzyme B). Other T cells mainly operate by releasing cytokines. Depending on the profile of secreted cytokines, these T cells can (i) elicit the typical lesions seen in delayed-type hypersensitivity (DTH) by attraction of mononuclear cells from the blood and the action of cytotoxic cytokines (like TNF-α) or (ii) offer help to B cells to differentiate into plasma cells for secretion of antibodies, or (iii) tolerate other cells. As a rule, CD8+ T cells act as CTL, whereas CD4+ T cells cause DTH or act as helper cells for B lymphocytes. Some CD8+ T cells, however, can also release lymphokines mediating DTH, and some CD4+ T cells have been demonstrated to exhibit CTL activity.

Graft rejection, GvHD and GvL are special manifestations of alloreactivity occurring in chimaeras (e.g. after allogeneic BMT). The general principles of alloreactivity outlined above are not suspended after allogeneic BMT. The setting for alloreactivity after BMT, however, is irregular, since tissues of different genetical origin coexist

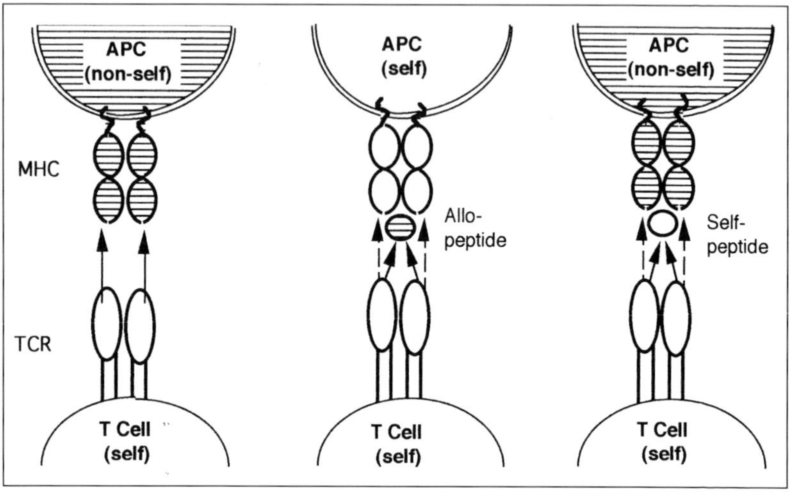

Fig. 5. The molecular basis of allorecognition. T cells may directly recognize epitopes on a non-self (mismatched) MHC (left). T cells may also recognize non-self-peptides presented by self-MHC (middle) or self-peptides presented by non-self-MHC (right). TCR-T-Cell receptor; MHC-major histocompatibility antigen; APC-antigen-presenting cell; self-▭; non-self-▤; binding sites-⟶. In case of GvHD, the T cells are of donor origin, and self means donor-self. In case of graft rejection, the T cells are of patient origin, and self means patients-self.

in one and the same organism ("chimaerism"). Consequently, "self" may be either "donor self" or "recipient self". After BMT, "self" T cells may (i) directly recognize epitopes on mismatched non-self HLA, (ii) recognize "non-self" peptides presented by "self" HLA molecules, or (iii) detect "self" peptides associated with non-self, mismatched HLA molecules as illustrated in figure 5. Since peptides may also be derived from mismatched HLA molecules, (ii) and (iii) include an "indirect pathway" for recognition of (mismatched) HLA molecules, whereas (i) is known as the "direct pathway" of HLA allorecognition.

2.4. Graft Rejection is Due to Alloreactivity Operating in HvG Direction

Graft rejection is caused by active destruction of the transplant by an immune reaction, whereas graft failure due to other causes (e.g. toxicity to stem cells from medication, viral infections, myelofibrosis) is not defined as graft rejection.

As demonstrated in clinical studies, graft rejection is associated with (i) the degree of genetic (HLA and minor transplantation antigen) disparity between the donor and the recipient, (ii) the quantity of patient's T cells surviving conditioning, (iii) the strategy of using T-cell depletion, i.e., removal of donor T cells from the graft, (iv) the quality of the posttransplant immunosuppressive therapy, and (v) the degree of alloimmunization induced by blood transfusions or pregnancies prior to BMT.

In humans, the exact pathomechanism of graft rejection is unknown. However, experimental work in animals suggests host T cells, B cells and NK cells (which have survived conditioning) to be involved. Host T (and B) cells are triggered by "non-self" major or minor histocompatibility antigens on the graft. The resulting HvGR takes several days to develop, and graft rejection is finally caused by the often combined activities of CTL, alloantibodies and/or increased concentrations of cytokines. In contrast, the HvGR mediated by NK cells starts within hours after transplantation. There is preliminary evidence that alloreactive NK cells have their target in HLA-C antigens. The interaction between NK-cell and self HLA molecules has been demonstrated to generate a negative signal, inhibiting cytolytic activities. Thus, in contrast to CTL, the absence of self class I on target cells might be crucial for NK-mediated killing.

High numbers of surviving, functionally active host T cells obviously increase the risk of graft rejection, whereas donor T cells exert a protective effect for the graft, presumably by inactivating or killing host T cells.

This observation is of great clinical relevance as evidenced by the following examples: (i) the use of T-cell depletion (removal of donor T cells from the graft in attempt to prevent GvHD), for example, increases the incidence of graft rejection from 1% to 10-30% in BMT with HLA-identical relatives; (ii) in BMT for malignant diseases, which require aggressive conditioning, a one-HLA locus mismatch (either one HLA-A or -B or -DR) is acceptable (in case of a related donor) since it does not significantly increase the risk of graft rejection; (iii) in BMT for severe aplastic anemia (SAA), however, which is generally prepared by less aggressive conditioning, a fully HLA-matched donor is requested by most transplanters.

2.5. GvHD is Due to Alloreactivity Operating in GvH Direction

Acute GvHD is a distinctive syndrome of dermatitis, hepatitis, and enteritis in recipients It develops within 100 days after allogeneic BMT and is due to immunological mechanisms operating in GvH direction. The occurrence of acute GvHD is linked to the condition that immunocompetent (virgin and experienced) donor T cells are transferred into a patient who shows disparity of transplantation antigens with the donor ("histocompatibility barrier") but is unable to reject the graft (as a consequence of conditioning or due to an underlying immunodeficiency disease).

The incidence of acute GvHD is associated with the following factors: (i) donor/recipient disparity of transplantation antigens; (ii) use of unmodified instead of T-cell-depleted marrow; (iii) alloimmunization of the donor by pregnancies or blood transfusions; (iv) sex mismatching, especially in case of female donors for male recipients; (v) advanced age of the recipient; (vi) highly aggressive conditioning protocols; (vii) low-dose posttransplant immunosuppression, and (viii) frequency of bacterial and viral infections after BMT (use of laminar airflow protection). As shown by a comprehensive retrospective analysis from Seattle, the risk of acute GvHD grades II-IV increased from 40% in BMT from genotypically HLA-identical siblings to over 80% in BMT from related donors with three HLA mismatches (1A, 1B, 1DR).

The precise pathogenesis of GvHD is unknown, but it might consist of the following chain of events: (i) Transplanted (virgin and experienced) and newly formed (virgin) "donor-anti-host" precursor T cells are activated by recognition of patient transplantation antigens on appropriate patient APC as described in paragraph 2.3. (ii) Once activated, precursor T cells show extensive clonal proliferation and finally differentiate into allospecific effector T cells in response to exogenous or endogenous cytokines. (iii) Effector T cells which have reached gut, liver, skin, and lung are triggered by patient antigens and cause tissue damages as detailed in paragraph 2.3.

Since sex-specific minor antigens (H-Y antigens on host cells) might increase the risk for acute GvHD, transplantation of male patients with female donors is avoided, if possible. Furthermore, infectious agents could act as triggers for acute GvHD possibly by sharing antigenic epitopes with gut epithelial cells, or by eliciting an inflammatory response, known to increase the expression of transplantation antigens.

Chronic GvHD is a more pleiotropic syndrome that develops after day 100 of allogeneic BMT. Also here, the exact pathomechanism is obscure. Some investigators take chronic GvHD as a late stage of acute GvHD due to minor alloantigen recognition. Others consider an "autoimmune-like" process and suggest a disorder of specific donor T-suppressor-cell functions to be operative. Although the clinical features of chronic GvHD and systemic autoimmune diseases do overlap considerably, an alloreactive component is certainly present, since in a large clinical study the incidence of chronic GvHD was found to be 33, 49, and 64% in BMT series using HLA-identical siblings, partially HLA-matched related donors, and fully matched unrelated donors, respectively.

2.6. The GvL Effect is a Beneficial Side of Alloreactivity

Allogeneic BMT is more effective in eradicating residual malignant cells than conventional chemotherapy, since (i) BMT allows the administration of more intensive chemotherapy and irradiation and (ii) immunocompetent cells of the graft exert an additional antineoplastic effect (GvL effect). Strong evidence for the existence of the GvL effect initially came from retrospective clinical studies on BMT performed for leukemia, indicating that the occurrence of GvHD was associated with a lower risk of relapse. Interestingly, recipients of syngeneic marrow (marrow from a monozygotic twin) who are not at risk for GvHD showed a significantly higher rate of relapse than recipients of HLA-identical allogeneic marrow. Furthermore, the incidence of relapse was found to be clearly higher after allogeneic BMT in patients who remained free from GvHD. T-cell depletion of donor marrow resulted in a decrease of GvHD incidence and an increase of relapse. However, allogeneic BMT may exert this beneficial effect even in the absence of GvHD, since recipients of allogeneic marrow without GvHD are also at a lower risk of relapse than are patients transplanted with syngeneic marrow. The GvL effect is mediated by donor CTL and NK cells. Leukemic cells are killed by direct cytolytic activity of these effector cells or by the release of cytokines (e.g., IL-2, TNF-α, IFN-γ). Potential targets for GvL are either normal host alloantigens or putative tumor-associated antigens. The central question for future developments is, whether it will become possible to separate the beneficial GvL effect of allogeneic BMT from GvHD by manipulation of the transplanted immune system.

2.7. Immune Reconstitution is the Gradual Replacement of the Widely Destroyed Immune System of the Recipient by the Donor Immune System

The conditioning regimen usually administered prior to BMT eliminates most cells of the host immune system. Hereby, a state of immunodeficiency is induced in the patient until immunity is gradually restored by grafted immunocompetent cells of donor origin. In case of BMT for congenital immunodeficiency syndromes, conditioning is generally not necessary and BMT is performed for the primary purpose to establish the donor immune system in the patient. The course of immune reconstitution, however, is basically the same in conditioned and primarily immunodeficient patients.

Immediately after BMT, some immunological functions are mediated by the small number of immunocompetent cells being present in the transfused marrow ("adoptive immune transfer"). Long-term immunological restoration against pathogens, however, seems to require exposure to antigens after BMT.

After transplantation, several factors govern the restoration of immunocompetent cells with regard to kinetics and biological functions: (i) the kind and dosage of immunosuppressive drugs administered posttransplant in order to prevent GvHD; prednisone, ciclosporin A, and antithymocyte globulin are all inhibitory for lymphocyte generation and function, and methotrexate adversely affects the proliferation of any cell; (ii) the occurrence and intensity of GvHD, which is immunosuppressive by itself; beside the skin, liver or gut, the lymphoid system is known to be a main target of the GvH reaction; (iii) the mass of residual thymic tissue, where the immature T cells undergo positive or negative selection; the thymus is naturally involuted in correlation to the recipient's age and, furthermore, may be damaged by radiation, cytotoxic drugs, and GvHD.

Hence, the time of restoration in number and cellular function varies considerably for the different components of the immune system. In the absence of chronic GvHD normal counts for neutrophils, monocytes, and total lymphocytes are achieved within 3-4 months after BMT from HLA-identical siblings. Whereas B cells quickly rise to, and CD8+ T cells as well as NK cells even rise above the normal range by 1 month posttransplant, total CD4+ T cells may be subnormal even 5 years after BMT. Thus, the normal CD4:CD8 ratio of 2 is found to be inverted in the long run posttransplant. Histologic studies make it hard to believe that the posttransplant thymus gives rise to a substantial amount of naive T cells. At 3-6 months after transplant most T cells are derived from the grafted mature T cells. In contrast to naive CD4+ T cells, naive CD8+ T cells might be generated de novo from marrow stem cells at an extrathymic side, since reconstitution of naive CD8+ T cells in terms of numbers is far better than of CD4+ naive T cells and does not correlate with the patient's age.

Newly derived neutrophils, monocytes, and NK cells seem to be able to function almost normally as soon as they are generated. The same might be true for mature and naive CD8+ (cytotoxic) T cells, but not for CD4+ T cells and not for B cells. Normal response of donor T lymphocytes to mitogens and antigens is not restored before 6–8 months after BMT, and the capacity of IL-2 secretion of CD4+ T cells may be suppressed even 12 months after BMT. Moreover, the T-cell repertoire (i.e., the recognition capabilities of the diverse antigens) may be restricted (i.e., oligoclonal) for up to several years following transplantation, and strongly overrepresented subsets of CD4+ T cells have been identified after BMT and were shown to exhibit donor-anti-host reactivity. With regard to B-cell function, the initially reduced serum levels of IgG and IgM recover within 9–14 months after BMT, whereas IgA serum concentrations normalize within 2 years. In patients without chronic GvHD almost normal immunological functions are restored within 1–2 years after BMT, whereas full competence is not achieved in the presence of chronic GvHD.

Active immunization with inactivated (killed) vaccines may generate a normal response as early as 1 year after BMT if chronic GvHD is absent. As a precaution, however, immunization with live vaccines is avoided even in healthy BMT patients for the rest of their lives.

2.8. A State of Tolerance between Donor and Recipient is Finally Achieved in All Surviving BMT Patients

The requirement of immunosuppressive treatment after allogeneic BMT may vary considerably from one patient to another. Finally, however, suppression can be discontinued in virtually all patients who survive BMT. The subsequent persistence of the graft in the absence of GvHD despite immune reconstitution (i.e., full reactivity of the transplanted immunocompetent donor cells against pathogens) indicates that a state of immunological tolerance has been achieved between the donor and the patient.

There are two current models for induction of self-tolerance during ontogenesis. According to the "self vs. non-self" recognition model of Harald von Boehmer, Basel Institute of Immunology, Switzerland, it is suggested that immature T cells arising from the marrow are deleted in the thymus if their T-cell receptors recognize "self antigens" with high affinity (negative selection), or are allowed to migrate to the periphery if expressing T-cell receptors that bind self peptides presented by the self HLA molecules with low affinity only (positive selection). Since these virgin T cells have not yet met all possible "self" antigens especially expressed on tissues other than thymus, this model postulates an additional "peripheral" mechanism of self-tolerance induction. A special toleration of B cells is not part of this model, since B-cell activation is thought to be dependent on help offered by non-tolerated T cells.

In contrast, the recent model of "dangerous vs. not dangerous" discrimination formulated by Polly Matzinger, National Institutes of Health, Bethesda, USA, suggests that T cells and B cells are clonally deleted if antigen encounter (signal 1) occurs in the absence of a 2nd signal called "costimulation" in case of T cells and "help" in case of B cells. Costimulation is offered by APCs, and help is provided by specific CD4+ (helper) T cells. Immature T cells are considered to be unable to accept signal 2 from any source; consequently, all thymocytes specific for antigens displayed in the thymus have to die. The costimulation requirements of mature T cells have already been outlined in paragraph 2.3. Thus, potential "autoreactive" virgin T cells are deleted in the periphery due to lack of appropriate costimulation as are autoreactive B-cell clones due to absence of adequate help from T cells.

Both theories mentioned above cannot be easily adopted to explain the induction of tolerance after BMT, since (i) transplanted marrow contains (beside immature and virgin T cells) also experienced T cells with anti-host reactivity; (ii) the host thymus might not be capable of tolerating virgin donor T cells, because it is involuted in adults and has generally been irradiated; (iii) alloantigens are imposed suddenly and in large quantity on immunocompetent cells (either of donor or recipient origin); (iv) immunocompetent cells encounter "non-self" HLA antigens associated with peptides derived from non-self and self antigens; (v) the host-type APCs within solid organs are gradually replaced by donor-type APCs within 1 year after BMT.

Even if there are no definitive data for humans, the following mechanisms for tolerance induction after BMT might be suggestive: (i) The life span of transplanted experienced donor T cells and residual experienced patient T cells almost certainly is finite. (ii) Newly formed (i.e., marrow graft-derived) T cells probably are tolerated in the patient's thymus for host-self and donor-self antigens. (After BMT the thymus basically remains of host origin, but can nevertheless also be repopulated by cells derived from the donor marrow.) (iii) Virgin donor T cells reactive against mismatched host HLA antigens might be tolerated as soon as professional donor APCs have replaced the professional host-type APCs. In this setting, all parenchymal cells of the patient continue expressing signal 1 (mismatched host alloantigens) to virgin donor T cells, but costimulation from professional APCs is no longer available.

3. Immunogenetic Bone Marrow Donor Search

H. Ottinger, H. Grosse-Wilde

This chapter will introduce readers to the current practice of clinical histocompatibility testing (tissue typing) and bone marrow donor search. Clinical histocompatibility testing is usually referred to as tissue typing. At present, tissue typing is confined to HLA typing of the marrow donor and the recipient. Notably, current tissue typing cannot eliminate the risk of graft rejection or GvHD due to minor histocompatibilty (mH) antigens, since routine techniques for assessment of mH differences between the donor and the patient are not (yet) available.

3.1. Methods for HLA Typing

3.1.1. HLA Class I and HLA Class II Serology

HLA serotyping, routinely performed as microdroplet lymphocytotoxicity test, relies on a panel of sera containing complement-fixing alloantibodies with specificity for antigenic epitopes on HLA class I and class II molecules. These sera are typically derived from individuals in whom the formation of specific HLA alloantibodies has been induced by pregnancies or blood transfusions. If a defined epitope is present on a tested cell, the corresponding HLA antibody will bind to the cell, the complement will be fixed, and consequently the cell will be killed. A dye which penetrates living cells will stain the dead cells and hereby indicate the presence of the epitope under evaluation (positive typing reaction). Class I typing (A,B,C) can readily be performed on unseparated (T + B) lymphocytes, whereas isolation of B cells is necessary for class II (DR, DQ) serotyping. Due to lack of high-quality antibodies, routine HLA-DP serotyping is not possible. HLA antigens as defined by serology are also called HLA specificities and most often do not correspond to a unique HLA allele, but to a group of different HLA alleles. Whereas some antisera detect supertypic ("broad", "public") HLA antigens, more specific antisera can subdivide these broad antigens into two or more split ("narrow", "private") antigens. For example, the two split antigens of the broad antigen HLA-B40 are named HLA-B60 and HLA-B61, and in tissue typing reports it is optional to add the broad antigen in parentheses after the typed narrow antigen, like HLA-B60(40). A major problem of

Table 1. HLA-A, -B, -C antigens/alleles identified for matching[a]

HLA-A	HLA-B	HLA-C
A1	B7	Cw1
A2	B703	Cw2
A203	B8	Cw3
A210	B13	Cw4
A3	B14	Cw5
A11	B65(14)	Cw6
A23(9)	B62(15)	Cw7
A24(9)	B63(15)	Cw8
A25(9)	B70	
A26(10)	B71(70)	
A29(19)	B75(15)	
A30(19)	B76(15)	
A31(19)	B77(15)	
A32(19)	B18	
A33(19)	B27	
A34(10)	B35	
A36	B37	
A43	B38(16)	
A66(10)	B39(16)	
A*6801(28)b	B60(40)	
A*6802(28)	B61(40)	
A*68VS(28)c	B41	
A*6901(28)	B42	
A74(19)	B*4402(12)	
	B*4403(12)	
	B*4404(12)	
	B*4405(12)	
	B45(12)	
	B46	
	B47	
	B48	
	B49(21)	
	B50(21)	
	B51(5)	
	B52(5)	
	B53	
	B54(22)	
	B55(22)	
	B56(22)	
	B*5701(17)	
	B*5702(17)	
	B*5801(17)	
	B59	
	B67	
	B73	

[a] The listed HLA-A und HLA-B antigens/alleles must be identified to permit a best match. Matching for HLA-C is preferred, but not mandatory. Designations preceded by an asteriks (*): alleles defined by DNA-based typing.

HLA serology is the cross-reactivity of the antisera used. Within their α_1 domain most HLA-B and some HLA-A molecules contain either the amino acid sequence N-L-R-I-A-L-R (Bw4 motif) or the sequence S-L-R-N-L-R-G (Bw6 motif). The Bw4 and Bw6 sequences are serologically detectable and are mutually exclusive epitopes. Since a given HLA-B specificity is associated with either Bw4 or Bw6 but not with both, the Bw4 and Bw6 motifs are of great help in HLA serology, e.g., to differentiate the broad antigen HLA-B12 into B44(Bw4) and B45(Bw6). A listing of the recognized HLA specificities is given in table 1. While HLA serology still is the cornerstone of routine HLA class I typing, HLA class II serotyping is gradually replaced by molecular genetic techniques.

3.1.2. Biochemical Typing of HLA Class I Antigens

One-dimensional isoelectric focusing (1D-IEF) gel electrophoresis is routinely available for typing of HLA-A and HLA-B and, in part, HLA-C antigens. Cellular glycoproteins including the HLA molecules are detergent-solubilized and submitted to gel electrophoresis and subsequent Western blotting. HLA class I molecules are visualized by developing the nitrocellulose membrane using a polyclonal antibody directed against a monomorphic part of HLA class I molecules, an alkaline phosphatase-coupled secondary antibody, and a dye. Due to their different amino acid sequences, most HLA-A and HLA-B alleles possess a characteristic isoelectric point and, therefore, can be identified by their typical banding pattern. Biochemical class I typing can detect further polymorphism of serologically defined HLA antigens. These biochemical subtypes of a given HLA specificity often correspond directly to the molecular genetically defined HLA alleles. Although 1D-IEF is a time-consuming procedure and cannot replace serological HLA typing, this method has been proven to be of great value to confirm serological class I typing results of patients and their prospective marrow donors.

3.1.3. Molecular Genetic (DNA) HLA Typing

Sequencing of the HLA alleles in all donor/recipient pairs is the most exact technique in order to identify the diversity of HLA at the genomic level. The nucleotide sequences of all currently recognized HLA class I and II alleles have been determined in research laboratories. Fully automated DNA sequencing is already used in some clinical laboratories to solve difficult typing problems. However, a DNA sequencing technique suitable for a large-scale routine application is not yet available. Fortunately, for the typing of individual HLA alleles it is not necessary to determine each nucleotide at its exact position. Genes or gene segments indicative for a given HLA allele can be identified by synthetic oligonucleotides (primers) and then selectively be amplified by means of the polymerase chain reaction (PCR). Based on this principle, DNA samples can be routinely analyzed for the presence or absence of particular HLA alleles by one of the following techniques: In the so-called PCR-SSO test, the gene segment corresponding to the most variable domain of a coding region (e.g., exon 2 for DRB1 genes) is PCR-amplified. A panel of sequence-specific oligonucleotide probes (SSOP) is then tested for hybridization with the amplified DNA. Hybridization of a particular SSOP signifies that the nucleotide sequence corresponding to this SSOP is present in the gene (exon 2). The presence of an individual HLA allele is finally identified by its characteristic hybridization pattern with the set of SSOP used. The use of allele-specific oligonucleotide probes instead of SSOP is also possible. A more straightforward technique is the use of sequence-specific primers for amplification (PCR-SSP). If an amplification occurs, the quantity of DNA will sharply rise in the test system, indicating that the particular allelic sequence is present.

DNA-based HLA typing techniques can be performed at a low("generic")-resolution or at a high-resolution level, according to the particular clinical needs (table 2). Whereas the latter precisely identifies the different alleles (e.g., DRB1*0101 or DRB1*0102), the former identifies narrow groups of alleles as does serology (e.g.,

Table 2. HLA-DRB1 alleles identified by (high-resolution) DNA-based typing[a]

DR1	DR2	DR3	DR4	DR7	DR8	DR9	DR10	DR11(5)	DR12(5)	DR13(6)	DR14(6)
DRB1*0101	DRB1*15011	DRB1*03011	DRB1*0401	DRB1*0701	DRB1*0801	DRB1*09011	DRB1*1001	DRB1*11011	DRB1*1201	DRB1*1301	DRB1*1401
DRB1*0102	DRB1*15012	DRB1*03012	DRB1*0402		DRB1*08021	DRB1*09012		DRB1*11012	DRB1*12021	DRB1*1302	DRB1*1402
DRB1*0103	DRB1*1502	DRB1*0302	DRB1*0403		DRB1*08022			DRB1*1102	DRB1*12022	DRB1*1303	DRB1*1403
DRB1*0104	DRB1*1503	DRB1*0303	DRB1*0404		DRB1*08031			DRB1*1103	DRB1*12031	DRB1*1304	DRB1*1404
	DRB1*1504	DRB1*0304	DRB1*0405		DRB1*08041			DRB1*11041	DRB1*12032	DRB1*1305	DRB1*1405
	DRB1*1601	DRB1*0305	DRB1*0406		DRB1*08042			DRB1*11042		DRB1*1306	DRB1*1406
	DRB1*1602		DRB1*0407		DRB1*0805			DRB1*1105		DRB1*1307	DRB1*1407
	DRB1*1603		DRB1*0408		DRB1*0806			DRB1*1106		DRB1*1308	DRB1*1408
	DRB1*1604		DRB1*0409		DRB1*0807			DRB1*1107		DRB1*1309	DRB1*1409
	DRB1*1605		DRB1*0410		DRB1*0808			DRB1*11081		DRB1*1310	DRB1*1410
	DRB1*1606		DRB1*0411		DRB1*0809			DRB1*11082		DRB1*1311	DRB1*1411
			DRB1*0412		DRB1*0810			DRB1*1109		DRB1*1312	DRB1*1412
			DRB1*0413		DRB1*0811			DRB1*1110		DRB1*1313	DRB1*1413
			DRB1*0414					DRB1*1111		DRB1*1314	DRB1*1414
			DRB1*0415					DRB1*1112		DRB1*1315	DRB1*1415
			DRB1*0416					DRB1*1113		DRB1*1316	DRB1*1416
			DRB1*0417					DRB1*1114		DRB1*1317	DRB1*1417
			DRB1*0418					DRB1*1115		DRB1*1318	DRB1*1418
			DRB1*0419					DRB1*1116		DRB1*1319	
			DRB1*0420					DRB1*1117			
			DRB1*0421					DRB1*1118			
			DRB1*0422					DRB1*1119			

[a] These HLA-DRB1 alleles must be identified to permit a best match (September 1995). Additional matching for HLA-DQB1 and DRB3, DRB4, and DRB5 alleles is not mandatory. However, when 2 or more donors equally matched for HLA-A, -B, and DRB1 are available, we will attempt to optimize matching for DQB1, DRB3, DRB4, and DRB5.

DRB1*010X, corresponding to the HLA-DR1 specificity). Molecular genetic HLA-DR,DQ,DP tissue typing is now widely used and has in part replaced serological HLA class II typing. For HLA class I antigens DNA-based typing of HLA-A alleles is already feasible; typing of HLA-B or -C alleles is still in its experimental stage but will be introduced in clinical testings during the next years.

3.1.4. Mixed Lymphocyte Culture (MLC) Test

This test can be taken as an in vitro assay for the primary allorecognition, since it detects the proliferation of T lymphocytes in response to alloantigens on B cells or monocytes from another individual. Routinely, the one-way MLC test is used, in which one part of peripheral blood mononuclear cells, either of the donor or of the recipient, is irradiated to inhibit their cell proliferation. The irradiated, alloantigen-expressing cells are called stimulator cells, and the untreated cells are called responder cells. To induce the donor-anti-recipient response (GvH direction), untreated donor cells are cocultured for 6 to 8 days with irradiated recipient cells. Vice versa, the recipient-anti-donor response (HvG direction) is tested by co-incubation of untreated recipient cells and irradiated donor cells. The degree of cell proliferation is measured by incorporation of ^{3}H- or ^{14}C-labelled thymidine into the DNA of the respective responder cells and expressed as relative response (RR) rates. If the RR exceeds 25%, the MLC test is scored as positive. As a rule, a positive MLC test indicates HLA class II disparity between the two individuals tested. It is well recognized that HLA-DR differences are responsible for most positive MLC tests. However, isolated HLA-DQ or HLA-DP differences can also induce T- cell proliferation under certain circumstances, and even mH antigen differences may sometimes cause a positive MLC test.

Although the MLC test cannot be considered any more to be the ultimate tool for HLA class II matching in marrow donor search, it still has its place as a final cellular cross-match for identified donor-recipient pairs, especially if more than one HLA-compatible donor candidate is available.

3.1.5. CTLp and HTLp Tests

There are recent reports that the number of circulating host-specific cytotoxic T-lymphocyte precursors (CTLp)and helper T-lymphocyte precursors (HTLp) are associated with the incidence of acute GvHD. Since the tests for CTLp and HTLp principally may also detect mH antigen differences, they can become of interest as predictive assays for GvHD in patients prior to BMT with HLA-identical donors. At present, both tests have not found a broader clinical application, and their predictive power for GvHD awaits to be established by multivariate statistical analysis.

3.1.6. Serological Cross-Matching

Pregnancies or blood transfusions may induce alloantibody formation. To detect patient alloantibodies specific for donor antigens prior to BMT, the capacity of the patient's serum to induce lysis of the donor's peripheral blood mononuclear cells is evaluated in the microdroplet lymphocytotoxicity test. This serological cross-matching is still practiced at our institution, but the "veto" to use a donor in case of a positive serological cross-matching is no longer absolute.

3.2. Types of Marrow Donor Search

There are 3 different types of bone marrow donor search, namely CFDS, EFDS and UMDS. Core family donor search (CFDS) is defined as search among the patient's siblings. For CFDS, it is routine at our institution to perform HLA class I serotyping and generic molecular genetic HLA-DR, DQ typing of the patient, his/her parents and all available siblings. The parents are included in this analysis to establish unequivocally the patient's HLA haplotypes. This principle is illustrated by the pedigree plot shown in figure 6. If an HLA-identical sibling donor has been identified, final MLC testing between the patient and this sibling is performed.

Extended family donor search (EFDS) refers to the search among other relatives than siblings. It is performed if (suitable) sibling donors are not available. Before EFDS starts, the patient's HLA haplotypes should have been identified by HLA class I and class II typing of the patient and his/her parents whenever possible. EFDS is then preferentially executed on that side of the family tree (maternal or paternal) where the less frequent patient HLA haplotype occurs and the more frequent patient haplotype is expected to be introduced by chance (marriage). EFDS is most effective among cousins, but half-siblings, aunts or uncles should also be tested. For EFDS, HLA class I serotyping is routinely performed in all possible donors, followed by generic DNA class II typing if appropriate, according to the match criteria for related donors outlined below. If a prospective donor is identified, confirmatory biochemical HLA class I and high-resolution HLA class II DNA typing of the donor and the patient are performed, followed by a final MLC test if appropriate.

Unrelated marrow donor search (UMDS) is bone marrow donor search among unrelated HLA-typed volunteers provided by national or foreign donor centers.

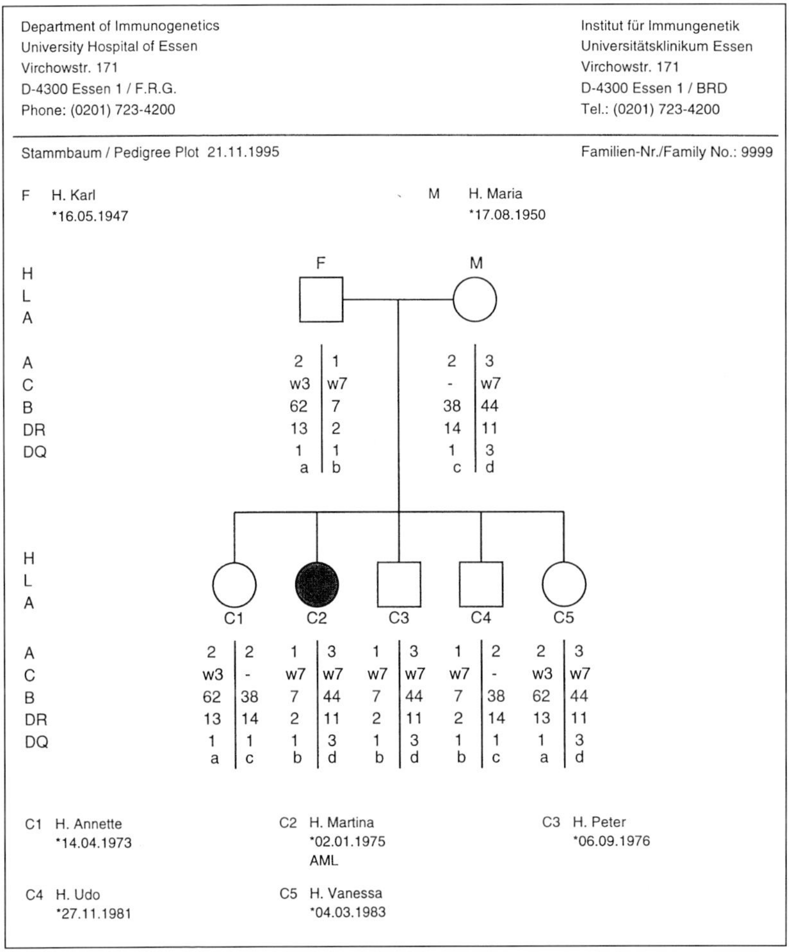

Fig. 6. A pedigree plot illustrating the mendelian inheritance of HLA haplotypes. F = father, M = mother; C1 – 5 = child No. 1–5; □ = male; ○ = female; ● = patient. The two paternal HLA haplotypes are named a and b, and the two maternal haplotypes c and d. The female patient C2 (AML) is HLA-genotypically identical with her brother C3, HLA-haploidentical with her brother C4 and her sister C5, but completely HLA-different from her sister C1.

UMDS is executed by an immunogenetic institution upon written request of the patient's primary physician (hematologist, oncologist or pediatrician) after (i) informed consent of the patient's side is given, (ii) a transplant center has approved the indication for a BMT with an unrelated donor, and (iii) the coverage of search costs is guaranteed. In preparation for the UMDS, the patient's HLA phenotype is confirmed by biochemical HLA class I typing and high-resolution DNA-based HLA class II (DR,DQ) typing. Additionally, the patient's HLA phenotype frequency in the general population is calculated. Presently (October 1994), about 2.2 million voluntary donors are available worldwide, including the 1.2 million donors of the US National Marrow Donor Program (NMDP), and 360,000 donors provided by German registries. The majority of these donors are typed only for HLA class I antigens. The most time-consuming process of UMDS is therefore to arrange HLA class II typing of numerous donors who are known to be class I identical with a given patient, until a volunteer is identified, who is also HLA class II matched. Subsequently, confirmatory biochemical class I and high-resolution DNA-based HLA class II typings of the prospective donor(s) are performed, followed by final MLC tests with the patient.

3.3. Strategy of Search

CFDS is the preferred type of search. It is both fast and cheap, and the clinical outcome of BMT with a genotypically HLA-identical sibling donor is the best. When CFDS has failed, our strategy is to perform EFDS next. EFDS generally is faster and less expensive than UMDS. Furthermore, in case of malignancy, the outcome of BMT from a partially HLA locus-mismatched related donor seems to be superior when compared to BMT from a fully HLA- matched unrelated donor. In urgent clinical settings, however, EFDS and UMDS should be run in parallel, since the most immediate donor is the best donor for this group of patients.

The HLA antigens/alleles that must be identified to permit a "best match" are listed in tables 1 and 2. (We are indebted to Effi W. Petersdorf, Program of Immunogenetics, Fred Hutchinson Cancer Research Center, Seattle, WA, USA, for her support in updating these tables.)

If a "best match" is unavailable for a patient with malignancy, our current criteria to accept partially HLA-matched donors are as follows:

In case of related donors, we accept 1 major HLA mismatch (1 HLA-A, -B or -DR disparity) or even 1 major HLA-A + 1 minor HLA-B mismatch in GvH direction, irrespective of the number of concomitant HLA mismatches in HvG direction and of the patient's age (0–55 years). In patients being homozygous at the HLA-A, -

B and -DR loci, for example, we proceed to transplant even with an HLA-haploidentical related donor (i.e., a donor exhibiting no mismatches in GvH, but 3 mismatches in HvG direction). In case of unrelated donors, our matching criteria are more strict: One HLA-minor antigen mismatch (HLA-A, -B or, -DR) is tolerated in patients ≤ 35 years, whereas a "best match" seems to be highly desirable in all patients > 35 years.

Our current definition for an "HLA class I major mismatch" is a "broad" HLA-A or HLA-B antigen difference between the donor and the recipient as defined by conventional serology (e.g., B7 vs. B16). In contrast, a "HLA class I minor mismatch" is a serological HLA-A or HLA-B "split" difference [e.g. B38(16) vs. B39(16)] or a difference in very closely related HLA-A or HLA-B alleles, which can only be identified by biochemical or molecular genetical methods. There are BMT units where mismatches for HLA-A or -B antigens belonging to a serologically "cross-reactive antigen group" (CREG) (e.g., A1 vs. A3 vs. A11 vs. A36) are regarded as a minor mismatch, but we have not yet adopted this policy. Our definitions for "HLA class II major and minor mismatches" are given in table 3.

Table 3. Definition of major versus minor HLA-DRB1 mismatches[a]

DR1	DRB1*0101–0104
DR15(2)	DRB1*1501–1504
DR16(2)	DRB1*1601–1606
DR17(3)	DRB1*0301; 0304; 0305
DR18(3)	DRB1*0302; 0303
DR4	DRB1*0401–0422
DR11(5)	DRB1*1101–1119
DR12(5)	DRB1*1201–1203
DR13(6)	DRB1*1301–1319
DR14(6)	DRB1*1401–1418
DR7	DRB1*0701
DR8	DRB1*0801–0811
DR9	DRB1*0901
DR10	DRB1*1001

[a] DR1–DR18 represent serologically defined specificities. Disparity for any of these specificities (e.g., DR1 vs. DR2) represents a major mismatch. Disparity for DRB1 alleles in each line represents minor mismatches, e.g., DRB1*0101 vs. *0102.

3.4. Success of Search

If these criteria are applied, a suitable donor is provided by CFDS for about 39%, by EFDS for an additional 6% of the patients. When focusing on (Caucasian) patients lacking a histocompatible related donor, the total overall UMDS success rate has meanwhile reached 70%, and an unrelated donor can be obtained for 50% of all UMDS patients within a period of 3 months after start of UMDS. Thus, the bone marrow donor search outlined above is finally successful for about 83% of all patients.

4. Conditioning Therapy

Prior to allogeneic BMT a pretreatment is necessary, which is also referred to as the conditioning therapy. This therapy has to be immunosuppressive and should "create space" for the graft. In patients with malignant diseases, the conditioning therapy should lead to complete eradication of the malignant cell clones. Over the years, a variety of conditioning protocols have been tested: the prevailing cytotoxic therapy in patients with severe aplastic anemia (SAA) is cyclophosphamide. For malignant diseases, the combination of cyclophosphamide and TBI is currently regarded as the standard conditioning regimen (table 4). The combination of high-dose busulfan in conjunction with cyclophosphamide, however, has been proven to be similar effective in patients with acute and chronic myeloid leukemia. Patients with intermediate- or high-grade malignant lymphomas are preferably treated by a combination of cytotoxic agents prior to autologous marrow or blood progenitor cell transplantation, because these patients have been frequently exposed to thoracic radiotherapy which may have led to lung tissue injury. Therefore, TBI-containing conditioning regimens are associated with an increased risk of toxic lung complications and should be omitted in these patients.

In advanced stages of hematopoietic malignant diseases, the standard conditioning regimens are often not sufficient to eradicate all malignant cells. For patients with SAA who have been sensitized through multiple blood transfusions, intensified immunosuppression by combining antilymphocyte globulins (ALG), antithymocyte globulins (ATG), total lymph node irradiation (TNI), or even TBI with cyclophosphamide have been recommended. When using exclusively cyclophosphamide in presensitized aplastic anemia patients, a higher rate of graft rejections has to be expected. In patients with leukemias, some centers have attempted to add etoposide, cytosine arabinoside or nitrosourea derivates to the standard TBI and cyclophosphamide regimen. However, toxicity of these escalated regimens appears to be generally increased, and there is currently no proof for a higher antitumor effect.

In the past, TBI delivered by linear accelerators or telecobalt sources with doses ranging between 8 and 10 Gy was generally performed in a single exposure. Currently, almost all transplant centers favor protocols using fractionated TBI with 1–3 daily fractions over several consecutive days. By using fractionated TBI schedules, a higher total dose can be delivered, since between radiation exposures some cell repair in healthy tissues can take place. In an attempt to decrease pulmonary toxicity of TBI, most centers shield the lungs to achieve a reduction of the lung dose by 10–20%. Similarly to escalated chemotherapeutic conditioning regimens, further

Table 4. Standard preparative regimens for allogeneic BMT

Severe aplastic anemia	
Cyclophosphamide	50 mg/kg/day on 4 consecutive days i.v.
± *antithymocyte globulin*	30 mg/kg/day on 3 consecutive days i.v.
Leukemias	
Cyclophosphamide	60 mg/kg/day on 2 consecutive days i.v.
+ *fractionated total-body irradiation*	total doses 10–14.5 Gy
or	
Cyclophosphamide	50 (60) mg/kg/day on 4 (2) consecutive days i.v.
+ *busulfan*	4 mg/kg/day on 4 consecutive days per os

dose escalation of TBI beyond a total dose of 12 Gy or hyperfractionated TBI schedules have no proven benefit with regard to patient outcome.

Fractionated TBI is clearly better tolerated than single-exposure TBI. Adverse reactions such as nausea and vomiting, chills and fever as well as parotic swellings, and diarrhea occur more frequently and with increased intensity in unfractionated TBI. Further, the majority of patients (about 80%) will develop cataracts within 3 to 5 years after unfractionated TBI, which frequently necessitates surgery. Whether dose fractionation will reduce the frequency of cataracts, or will only delay its onset, is currently uncertain. Gastrointestinal mucositis and alopecia which are caused by the conditioning treatment are reversible. As a consequence of TBI, females usually develop gonadal insufficiency, which nearly always results in sterility. In males, oligo-azoospermia is the rule. However, after single-agent cyclophosphamide conditioning in women with aplastic anemia, pregnancies resulting in the birth of healthy children have been repeatedly reported. In children receiving TBI, disturbances of growth and sexual development are prominent problems. These might be greatly reduced by using fractionated radiation.

As part of the conditioning treatment preceding marrow transplantation, TBI has to be supralethal, and is thus inevitably associated with adverse effects on many organ systems. Life-threatening complications like interstitial pneumonia, hepatic veno-occlusive disease and cardiac insufficiency are frequent toxic complications of this very intensive therapy. Different factors influence the efficacy and toxicity of TBI. These include, among others, the total radiation dose, the fractionation schedule, the homogeneity of radiation, the radiation source, the position of the patient during irradiation, and the type of lung shielding. Complex physical and radiobiological interactions make comparisons between centers difficult. For comparative analyses on toxicity and efficacy of TBI it is definitely not sufficient to take only the TBI doses into account.

High-dose cyclophosphamide infusions can lead to toxic hemorrhagic cystitis. This can be generally prevented by administration of mesna (Uromitexan®) and forced diuresis. To prevent nausea and vomiting, potent and combined antiemetic agents are mandatory. Busulfan in high doses can lead to convulsions, and prophylactic administration of anticonvulsants is therefore recommended.

5. Technique of Marrow Harvest

Harvesting marrow for use in bone marrow transplantation (fig. 7) is performed in a sterile operation room under general or peridural anesthesia, using multiple needle aspirations in the area of the superior iliac crest. The procedure lasts about 45–90 min. In order to reduce the amount of contaminating peripheral blood cells, small volumes of 3–6 ml should be aspirated from each of several locations. A total volume of 600–1,600 ml is usually needed, depending upon the recipient's body weight. The graft should contain at least between 2×10^8 and 4×10^8 nucleated cells per kg of the recipient's body weight. For autologous marrow transplantation an amount of 1×10^8 cells per kg is sufficient. The aspirated marrow cells are suspended in tissue culture medium containing heparin. After collection, the marrow cell suspension is centrifuged and filtered to remove fat, bone particles, and cell clumps. The marrow cells are then transfused into a central venous catheter using standard blood transfusion sets. In some centers each individual aspirate is pressed through a filter into a container. The total volume is then given to the patient without further centrifugation and filtration.

If the major ABO blood groups are incompatible between the recipient and the donor, the erythrocyte content of the graft has to be reduced to avoid hemolytic reactions. This can be achieved by different cell separation techniques, such as the "buffy-coat" technique, or by using blood cell separators. Alternatively, the recipient's isohemagglutinins can be reduced by plasma exchange. If the recipient's isohemagglutinin titer is low, the isohemagglutinins can be neutralized with repeated transfusions of the donor's ABO blood group. The unseparated marrow cell suspension can then be carefully transfused. Major ABO incompatibility sometimes can result in transient signs of hemolysis, or may lead to persistent anemia. Long-term suppression of erythropoiesis can be treated by plasmapheresis or transfusion of incompatible red blood cells, which are capable of adsorbing the recipient's isohemagglutinins.

As a prerequisite, marrow donors should be in normal good health. Two to 3 weeks prior to the procedure, one whole blood unit should be taken from the marrow donor. This is stored until retransfusion during marrow harvest.

The marrow donor should not be given foreign blood products. During marrow harvest the donor's white blood cells and platelets can increase to above the normal range. Occasionally, anemia caused by marrow donation can last a few days or even weeks. This is especially true when the marrow donor is also the recipient's blood donor. The principle risks for the donor are those inherent in any general anesthesia.

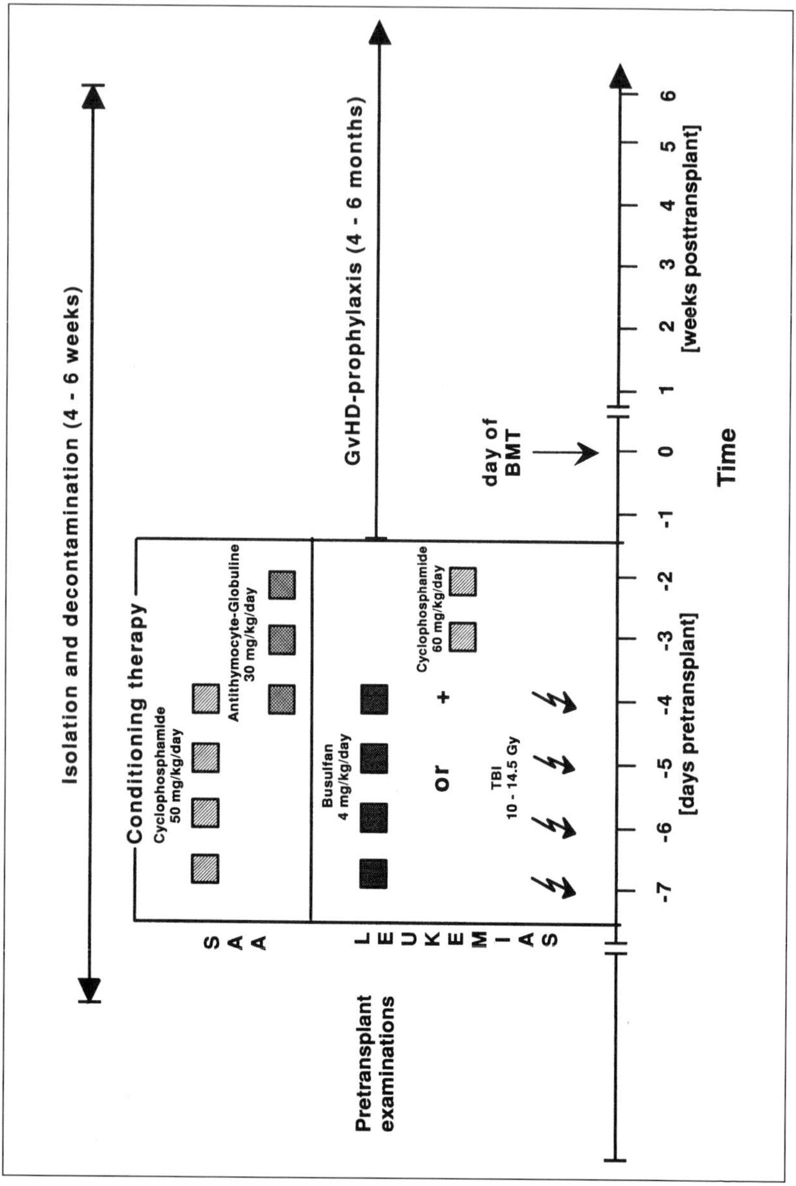

Fig. 7. Scheme of the time course in BMT.

A few cases of life-threatening complications associated with the marrow harvest procedure have been also reported.
The puncture areas usually remain painful for a few days. In rare instances, pain of these areas may persist for weeks or infections in the puncture may occur. Generally, the marrow donor can be discharged from the hospital on the day after marrow harvest. Since the marrow donor is also the ideal blood donor for the respective patient during the first weeks after transplantation between relatives, he or she should be prepared to donate blood during this time period. Prior to transplantation, however, the prospective marrow donor or any other family member should under no circumstances be used as blood donor for the patient. This can result in specific sensitization of the recipient against non-shared histocompatibility antigens, and may in turn lead to an increased risk of graft rejection.

Currently, sibling donors or donors from the extended family are considered first. In patients lacking a histocompatible marrow donor within his/her family, marrow transplantations using matched volunteer-unrelated marrow donors are increasingly performed. This approach is still regarded as experimental.

6. Clinical Course after Allogeneic Bone Marrow Transplantation

6.1. Supportive Therapy

At the time of marrow transplantation, the patient's peripheral white blood cell and platelet counts have already reached low levels due to the conditioning treatment. To prevent bleeding, platelet levels should be kept above $20 \times 10^9/l$ by giving platelet concentrates, preferably prepared by blood-cell separators. During the phase of marrow aplasia, a minimum of three platelet transfusions per week is usually necessary, and in certain clinical situations the platelet support may be substantially higher.

During the phase of marrow aplasia induced by the conditioning regimen, most patients develop febrile episodes and infections, irrespective of all preventive measures. Since these infections can be potentially life-threatening, fever should always be treated immediately with broad-spectrum systemic bactericidal antibiotics, without awaiting cultural proof of the infectious agent. Generally, double or triple combinations including aminoglycosides, penicillins or cephalosporins are recommended for the first-line treatment of suspected bacterial infections (table 5). It is important that these bactericidal combinations cover the gram-negative as well as the gram-positive bacterial microflora. Gram-positive bacterial infections have become an increasing problem in granulocytopenic patients during recent years. Therefore, vancomycin is now more frequently included in combined antibiotic regimens.

Despite high dose antibiotic combination therapy, patients seldom become afebrile in the early phase of marrow aplasia. However, discontinuation of therapy is not advisable, even when fever of unknown origin (FUO) is suspected. In all FUO situations, systemic antimycotic treatment has to be considered. Even if a mycotic infection is not unequivocally proven, antimycotic treatment should nevertheless be initiated early if there is any evidence or suspicion for an invasive fungal infection. In general, intravenous amphotericin B in combination with 5-fluorocytosin is the first-line therapy for fungal organ infections (table 5). Due to better tolerance, amphotericin B is often given as a continuous intravenous infusion over 12–24 h. Whether liposomal preparations of amphotericin B are more effective in the treatment of invasive fungal infections after marrow transplantation has currently not been proven by comparative studies.

Herpes simplex or varicella zoster virus infections have to be treated by parenteral acyclovir therapy (table 5).

Table 5. Systemic antimicrobial regimens in transplant patients

Empirical antibacterial therapy
Ureido-penicillins (cephalosporin) + penicillinase-resistant penicillin (Vancomycin) + aminoglycoside
Alternative, commonly used agents for combined antibiotic regimens:
Imipenem, Fosfomycin, Quinolones, Rifampicin, Teicoplanin
Antimycotic therapy
Amphotericin B ± 5-fluorocytosine
Alternative agents:
Fluconazol (Candida species), Itraconazol (Aspergillus species?), liposomal amphotericin preparations
Antiviral therapy
Acyclovir (varicella-zoster virus, herpes simplex virus)
Ganciclovir ± hyperimmonoglobulins (CMV)

In earlier years some centers used to give granulocyte transfusions as prophylaxis for infections. Since viruses may be transmitted with granulocyte transfusions, this supportive measure is no longer performed. In seronegative patients who receive transplants from seronegative marrow donors, cytomegalovirus transmission can effectively be prevented by exclusively using blood products from cytomegalovirus antibody-negative blood donors. All blood products, such as platelet concentrates, packed red cells or whole-blood transfusions, should be irradiated with 15-25 Gy in order to eliminate immunocompetent lymphocytes, which may induce transfusion-associated acute GvHD. In this dose range of irradiation, viability and function of red blood cells, platelets and granulocytes are not essentially impaired.

Generally, peripheral blood cell counts begin to rise during the 2nd or 3rd week after transplantation. This usually results in a rapid control of infections. Aside from febrile infections, patients in the phase of marrow aplasia often suffer from severe oral mucositis, nausea and vomiting, and diarrhea. Parenteral nutrition using central venous catheters is commonly used to avoid malnutrition. Sustained venal access is best guaranteed by Hickman catheters, which are subcutaneously implanted and fixed by a plastic cuff at the catheter exit site. This type of catheter can be left in place for several weeks. Of course it has to be removed if catheter infections develop or are even suspected. It is important to be aware that gram-positive cocci can become embedded in the plastic material of venous catheters.

The application of hematopoietic growth factors – especially granulocyte colony-stimulating factors – after allogeneic or autologous marrow or blood progenitor cell transplantation, intended to accelerate posttransplant granulocyte recovery, cannot be generally recommended. Aside from economical considerations, the clinical benefit of this supportive measure has not been documented for the majority of transplant settings so far.

6.2. Gnotobiotic Measures

Thorough prophylactic precautions against infections are particularly important in allogeneic BMT patients. Preferably, patients should be treated in an environment which is nearly or completely germ-free. The patient's bacterial and fungal microflora should be eliminated or suppressed by oral nonabsorbable antibiotics and antimycotics (table 6). In addition, a daily bath in disinfectant solutions is recommended to deplete the skin microflora. Since fungal intestinal pathogens may thrive after bacterial decontamination, mycotic decontamination should be started a few days prior to the initiation of bacterial decontamination. Decontamination and isolation measures should be continued until the patient is discharged from hospital. This is justified by the assumption that decontamination measures prevent or diminish endogenous bacterial and mycotic infections. Further, experimental and clinical evidence suggests that effective gastrointestinal decontamination can abolish or mitigate acute GvHD. For these reasons it is our policy to keep patients under strict isolation and decontamination until day 35 posttransplant. Of course, the efficacy of decontamination and isolation has to be constantly monitored by taking regular surveillance cultures, and it is not uncommon that these cultures provide an early identification of organisms responsible for infections. It is well established that most infections of granulocytopenic patients are caused by germs of the patient's endogenous intestinal microflora. As prophylaxis for exogenous infections, everything in the patient's room should be disinfected or sterilized. This also includes patient's oral intakes, in order to maintain total gastrointestinal decontamination. Laminar airflow units and rooms with air filtration have proven to be especially effective in prevention of infections (fig. 8).

6.3. Complications

After allogeneic BMT, immunosuppressive therapy is needed to prevent acute GvHD. Currently, the combination of a short course of methotrexate and continuous ciclosporin A represents the standard immunopharmacologic regimen. Unlike the situation after solid-organ transplantation, the immunoprophylaxis needs not to be continued indefinitely and is generally necessary over 6 to 12 months after the

Table 6. Measures for prevention of infection

Isolation in a germ-free environment
Skin disinfection
Gastrointestinal decontamination using nonabsorbable antibiotics and antimycotics
Autoclaved food
Cotrimoxazole or pentamidine prophylaxis against *Pneumocystis carinii*
Blood product substitution using CMV antibody-negative donors in seronegative donor/recipient combinations
CMV hyperimmunoglobulin prophylaxis (?)
Acyclovir prophylaxis

transplantion. If acute or chronic GvHD develops, immunosuppressive therapy will have to be intensified and given for longer periods.

Beside the susceptibility toward infections and bleeding, other complications like interstitial pneumonia and hepatic veno-occlusive disease may develop in the early posttransplant period. Both complications reflect, at least in part, transplant-related toxicities. In the pathogenesis of posttransplant interstitial pneumonia, the cytomegalovirus is the leading pathogen. For prophylaxis of *Pneumocystis carinii* pneumonia, most centers use oral cotrimoxazol or pentamidine aerosol inhalations before and after allogeneic transplantation. To prevent or ameliorate cytomegalovirus disease, prophylactic ganciclovir and/or foscavir are currently being investigated. Prophylactic acyclovir, which may also be active in suppressing cytomegalovirus disease, is frequently used to prevent herpes simplex reactivation.

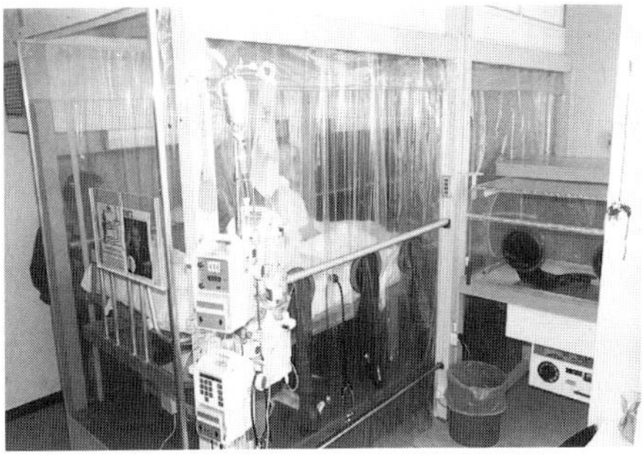

Fig. 8. Laminar-airflow isolation unit (downstream) (Pielkenrood-Vinitex b.v. Assendelft, The Netherlands).

By following the above mentioned guidelines of patient care, as well as measures for the prevention and treatment of infections or immunologic complications, the critical early posttransplant phase of pancytopenia can successfully be bridged in the vast majority of patients, and treatment-related fatalities in the early course after allogeneic BMT have become uncommon. However, a number of life-threatening complications remain after complete hematopoietic reconstitution.

When BMT is successful, the patient retains a stable hematopoietic chimaeric status of donor-type hematopoietic cells throughout his or her life. It has also been shown that osteoclasts, hepatic and alveolar macrophages as well as Langerhans cells are derived from the transplanted marrow cells.

Hematopoietic chimaerism can be proven by individual-specific markers, like sex chromosomes, red blood cell groups, immunoglobulin allotypes, and polymorphic enzymes. More recently, molecular biology techniques like variable number of tandem repeats analysis (VNTR) offers enhanced sensitivity to demonstration of chimaerism. Occasionally, a mixed chimaerism can be observed in which hematopoietic donor and recipient cells exist side by side. If residual hematopoietic recipient cells are present after allogeneic BMT performed for leukemia, this may indicate an increased risk of leukemic recurrence. The molecular detection of minimal residual disease by the genome sequence-specific amplification of the bcr/abl protooncogene using the PCR has already emerged as an important tool for early diagnosis of recurrent disease in patients with CML after allogeneic BMT. In very rare but remarkable cases, investigation of the chromosomes has proven that the donor graft cells underwent leukemic transformation. Most leukemic relapses after BMT, however, originate from residual malignant cells of the transplant recipient.

In the 1st year after BMT, patients generally have an increased susceptibility to infections due to persisting immunodeficiency. Infections caused by herpesviruses are especially frequent, but also less common opportunistic infections like toxoplasmosis or tuberculosis may be observed. Interstitial pneumonia occurs most frequently within the first 6–10 weeks following transplantation. The development of acute GvHD is restricted to the first 70 days posttransplant, but patients remain at risk for de novo onset or secondary chronic GvHD up to 2 years after transplantation. Thereafter, relapse of leukemia constitutes the predominant complication. This usually occurs within the first 3 years posttransplant. Nevertheless, in very rare instances relapses up to 6 years after transplantation have been observed.

Late complications include cataracts, sterility, and growth disorders in children. As mentioned above, the incidence of cataracts and growth disorders in children has been greatly reduced by using fractionated TBI.

The risk of secondary malignancies appears low at the moment. However, observation times of more than 20 years in only a few patients preclude definite conclusions regarding the risk of this late complication.

7. Indications for Allogeneic Bone Marrow Transplantation and Clinical Results

The broadly accepted major indications for allogeneic BMT are summarized in table 7.

7.1. Severe Aplastic Anemia

Severe aplastic anemia (SAA) is a syndrome characterized by insufficient production of blood cells. Dyshematopoiesis can vary in intensity and clinical progression. The etiology of SAA often remains unclear. Exposure to radiation, chemicals, medications as well as viral infections like hepatitis may play a causative role or promote aplastic anemia. Damage to the hematopoietic stem cells or to the hematopoietic microenvironment are relevant factors in the pathogenesis of aplastic anemia. Immunologic factors can also disturb the stem cell potential, for example by activation of suppressor lymphocytes or by cytotoxic antibodies.

Aplastic anemia is characterized by pancytopenia and hypocellularity of the bone marrow. SAA is defined by absolute granulocyte counts below $0.5 \times 10^9/l$, platelet counts below $20 \times 10^9/l$, and reticulocyte counts below 10‰. Patients with this condition have a mortality rate of 70–80%, and death usually occurs within the first 6 months after the diagnosis of SAA.

Conventional therapy for aplastic anemia consists of blood product substitution and antibiotic treatment in infected patients. Many authors have reported on the positive effects of androgens. Prospective studies, however, were not able to definitely prove the therapeutic effectiveness of androgens. In contrast, immunosuppressive therapy has been successful in some patients. Corticosteroids, antilymphocyte sera (ALS), antithymocyte globulins (ATG), ciclosporin and cyclophosphamide have all been used. In studies involving ALS and ATG, the hematopoiesis in about 50% of patients improved, and responding patients became independent of transfusion. However, often only partial remissions can be attained. Relapse of marrow aplasia after initially successful therapy is not uncommon.

The idea of using the donor's healthy bone marrow to correct the patient's defective stem cell system is enticing. Since only a minority of patients has a syngeneic or allogeneic marrow donor, and in light of the risks inherent in BMT, the development of in vitro tests that predict response to conventional immunosuppressive therapy should receive greater attention. BMT after failure of ALS therapy has only a re-

Table 7. Established indications for allogeneic BMT

Malignant hematologic diseases
Acute myeloid leukemia
Acute lymphoblastic leukemia
Chronic myeloid leukemia
Myelodysplastic syndromes with leukemic transformation
Acute osteomyelofibrosis
Nonmalignant diseases
Severe aplastic anemia
Severe combined immunodeficiency
Thalassemia major
Fanconi's anemia

duced chance of success, because patients who received multiple transfusions have an increased risk of graft rejection. Furthermore, complications like bleeding and infections are more likely after protracted illness.
In selecting patients for BMT, three points are decisive:

1. Severity of disease;
2. Availability of a histocompatible donor;
3. Age of the patient.

The causes of SAA are of secondary importance. However, in Fanconi's anemia it should be remembered that these patients have a reduced DNA repair capacity. Therefore, Fanconi's anemia patients are at a greater risk of developing toxic organ complications after chemo- or radiotherapy, which has also to be considered in immunosuppressive regimens prior to BMT. Pancytopenia in the course of paroxysmal nocturnal hemoglobinuria can also be successfully treated by BMT, although secondary organ siderosis and sensitization as a consequence of multiple blood transfusions may cause serious problems in the clinical posttransplant course.

Most centers agree that aplastic anemia patients under the age of 50 years who have an HLA-identical sibling donor should receive BMT as soon as possible. Immunosuppressive treatment as first-line therapy is recommended when only a partially histocompatible family or a matched unrelated donor is available, or in elder patients. After failure of conventional therapy, BMT with a partially matched related donor or with an HLA-phenotypically identical unrelated donor should be considered (fig. 9).

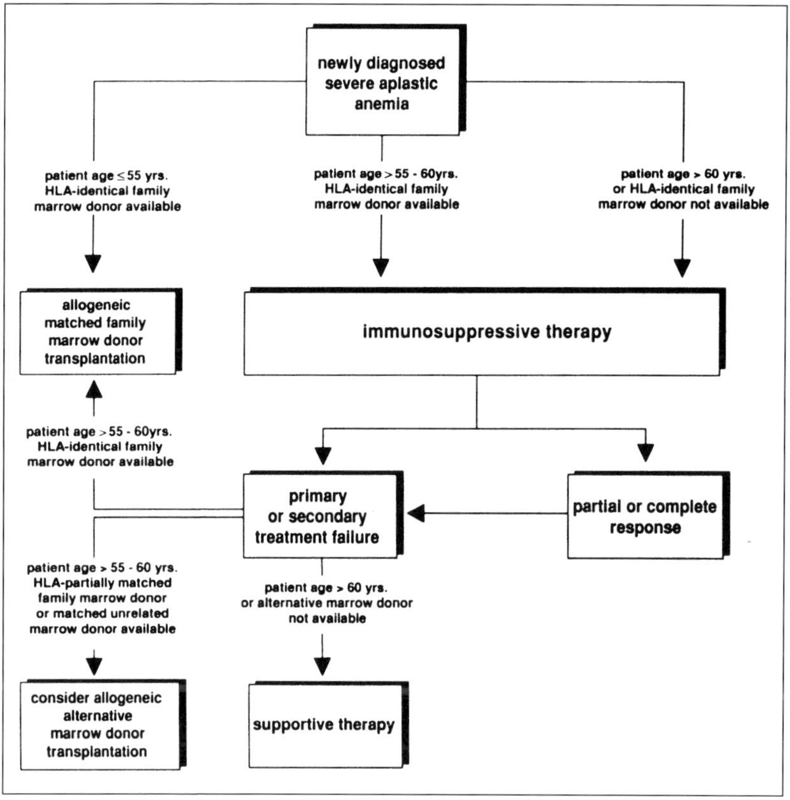

Fig. 9. Decision organigram for the indication of allogeneic BMT in patients with severe aplastic anemia.

7.1.1. Preparative Measures

Once the diagnosis of SAA has been established, indication for BMT should immediately be discussed with the respective transplant center, if a suitable marrow donor has been identified. It is particularly important to avoid any blood transfusions in patients with aplastic anemia who are potential transplant candidates. Under no circumstances, however, should family members be used as blood donors in these patients, because the resulting sensitization against minor histocompatibility antigens would increase the risk of graft rejection. Retrospective analyses have clearly demonstrated that the success of transplantation is directly connected with the number of blood transfusions given earlier than 48 h to the initiation of immunosuppressive conditioning. Best results were obtained in untransfused patients. The risks of transfusion-induced sensitization, as well as of bleeding and infectious complications, can be greatly reduced by performing transplantation as early as possible.

Supportive measures for transplant recipients should be planned with great care. For platelet substitution, concentrates prepared by blood cell separators should be used whenever possible. If the patient develops fever or other signs of infection, the same diagnostic and therapeutic principles apply as for immunodeficient neutropenic patients receiving chemotherapy. Bacteriologic cultures of blood, oral washings, urine, feces and skin swabs should immediately be taken, and an empirical systemic combined bactericidal therapy should be initiated without delay. Antibiotics can be adjusted later according to laboratory results. For empirical therapy, combinations of synthetic penicillins or cephalosporins and aminoglycoside have proven successful. If systemic fungal infection is suspected, parenteral therapy with antimycotic antibiotics has to be considered early. Prophylaxis of mycotic infections using oral antimycotics is generally recommended in these patients.

7.1.2. Conditioning and Transplantation

Prior to allogeneic BMT, the recipient's immune system must be efficiently suppressed to ensure marrow engraftment. Cyclophosphamide, applied intravenously in 4 consecutive daily doses of 50 mg/kg body weight, has proved effective. In the past, the Seattle group recommended transfusions of donor buffy-coat cells 1 day prior to the start of the immunosuppressive treatment with cyclophosphamide. The idea behind this was to stimulate the recipient's immunocompetent lymphocytes with donor-cell antigens, which in turn should result in an increased susceptibility of these cells toward the cytotoxic effects of cyclophosphamide. This theoretical advantage, however, could not be confirmed in clinical practise, and this procedure is not used any more.

Hemorrhagic cystitis, a well-established adverse effect of cyclophosphamide therapy, can effectively be prevented by uroprotection with mesna in combination with forced diuresis. For prophylaxis of nausea and vomiting induced by cyclophosphamide, systemic antiemetics should be initiated early.

If the patient has been sensitized due to multiple transfusions, it will be necessary to intensify the immunosuppressive pretreatment by additional total lymph node irradiation or application of ATG. TBI should not be used in aplastic anemia patients because of its substantial acute toxicity and its late adverse effects.

Intravenous administration of the graft should follow within 24–48 h after the last course of cyclophosphamide. The graft should contain a minimum of $3–4 \times 10^8$ nucleated cells per kg of the recipient's body weight. Multitransfused patients in particular, who receive a graft with a lower cell quantity, have an increased risk of graft rejection. If the graft cell content is below 3×10^8/kg body weight, peripheral buffy-coat donor blood transfusions on the first 5 days after transplantation may be considered. The Seattle group demonstrated that the use of donor buffy-coat transfusions improved allogeneic marrow engraftment in these situations. However, it became apparent that this is achieved at the expense of an increased risk for the development of GvHD.

If an identical twin donor is available, transplantation can be attempted without any immunosuppressive pretreatment. If the first transplant does not result in permanent hematopoietic reconstitution, the transplantation can be repeated after conditioning with cyclophosphamide.

7.1.3. Clinical Results

The clinical results of bone marrow transplantation in patients with SAA have steadily improved over the past 15 years. The longest period of observation has now reached 20 years. Initially, about 45% of patients could be cured. Now the chance of cure has reached 70–80%, assuming that transplantation is performed early in the course of disease and the donor is an HLA- and MCL-identical family member.

The Seattle group reported on 50 HLA-identical sibling marrow transplants in patients with aplastic anemia, who had not received blood transfusions until 48 h prior to the first cyclophosphamide application. The survival probability of these patients was 82%, with an observation time of 3–15 years. Graft rejection was very infrequent. In contrast, about 30% of patients who had received multiple transfusions rejected their grafts.

Besides rejection, acute and chronic GvHD are predominant predictors of survival. According to the Seattle experience, the incidence of grades II-IV acute GvHD was 55% when the donor was an HLA-identical family member and methotrexate was used as immunoprophylaxis. In a more recent trial, which investigated the combination of methotrexate and ciclosporin, the incidence of moderate to severe acute GvHD was reduced to 18%. This combination did not reduce the occurrence of chronic GvHD, which manifested in 40–50% of patients.

The most recent patient cohort from Seattle was treated with a combination of cyclophosphamide and ATG prior to allogeneic BMT from HLA-identical sibling donors, and received a short course of methotrexate and ciclosporin A for the prevention of acute GvHD. In this patient group, which included a high proportion of patients failing conventional immunosuppressive therapy and of multitransfused patients, survival was in the range of 90%. This figure compared favorably to a similar patient group which received only cyclophosphamide as pretransplant immunosuppressive conditioning.

A study from Seattle further demonstrated that gnotobiotic measures, including oral decontamination and isolation in laminar-airflow rooms, reduced the incidence of acute GvHD and improved the survival of patients with aplastic anemia.

The International Bone Marrow Transplant Registry (IBMTR) in Milwaukee (USA) analyzed the results of 455 patients with SAA, who had received an allogeneic graft from an HLA-identical family member. Of 163 patients treated between 1978 and 1980, 47 (±9)% survived. In 292 patients treated since 1981, survival was 63 (±7)% at 4 years after transplantation. According to the results of the IBMTR, transplantation in sex-matched donor/recipient combinations is more successful than in sex-mismatched combinations (63 (±6)% vs. 45 (±9)%).

Interstitial pneumonia, previously one of the most common causes of death in leukemia patients, occurs much less frequently in aplastic anemia patients. This observation may also be taken as indirect evidence that TBI, as the major component of conditioning regimens in leukemia patients, increases the risk of interstitial pneumonia. In the IBMTR analysis, aplastic anemia patients who did not receive radiotherapy as part of the conditioning had an incidence of interstitial pneumonia in the range of 10%, in contrast to a 30% incidence in leukemia patients. In about 80% of patients with interstitial pneumonia, this complication was fatal, and in 40% of interstitial pneumonia cases cytomegalovirus could be detected. An additional significant risk factor for the development of interstitial pneumonia was the presence of severe acute GvHD. Further, the type of immunoprophylaxis for acute GvHD proved to be a significant risk factor for interstitial pneumonia, which occurred less frequently in patients who received exclusively ciclosporin A as compared to patients who weekly received methotrexate.

Cataracts, disorders in endocrine functions, and growth disorders in children, often observed after TBI, are rare in aplastic anemia patients. Reports of healthy children born to female patients after allogeneic BMT for aplastic anemia are now becoming more common. Up to now, the rate of secondary malignancies does not seem to be increased, although the observation period is still rather short.

7.2. Leukemias

The therapeutic principle behind bone marrow transplantation for acute or chronic leukemia is to eradicate the patient's malignant hematopoiesis with high-dose cytotoxic treatment and replace the eradicated marrow function by bone marrow of a suitable donor. Although conventional chemotherapy for acute leukemias has considerably improved within recent years, the majority of adult patients, as well as a high proportion of children with acute leukemias and unfavorable prognostic factors, still relapse and subsequently die of their disease. It can be assumed that many of these patients would survive, and even be cured, if higher doses of chemotherapy could be tolerated. Prolonged myelosuppression and organ toxicities, however, set narrow limits for chemotherapy. Since the myelosuppressive effects of high-dose therapy can be counteracted by BMT, treatment protocols with higher curative potential become applicable.

At the very beginning, BMT was exclusively used in refractory end stages of leukemic diseases. As could be expected, the results were not satisfactory, even though a small proportion of patients became long-term survivors or were cured. Since the concept of BMT was first experimentally tested in irradiated animals, it is no wonder that TBI became an important element of conditioning regimens for allogeneic BMT in humans. For several years, TBI was delivered in a single dose. Currently, most centers use fractionated irradiation schedules, which allow the application of higher doses without increased toxicity. TBI as the sole mode of pretreatment, however, proved to be not sufficiently antileukemic. Therefore the Seattle group added cyclophosphamide, given intravenously 4 or 5 days prior to TBI. This combination of TBI and cyclophosphamide still remains the standard protocol for comparison to other conditioning regimens. Conditioning programs which include additional cytotoxic drugs have usually proven to be too toxic and thus have had to be abandoned. It should, however, be noted that these negative experiences involved predominantly end-stage patients who had been intensively pretreated and were often in poor general condition. In addition, a large leukemic cell burden with resistant clones must be assumed in such patients. Since marrow transplantation is now preferably performed in early disease stages, more intensive conditioning regimens may be more suitable. It appears therefore appropriate to reinvestigate whether the standard conditioning regimen can be improved by the addition of cytotoxic agents.

Conditioning regimens not using TBI have also been described. The combination of high- dose busulfan and cyclophosphamide, which was pioneered by the Baltimore group, has been found to be particularly effective in acute and chronic myeloid leukemia.

7.2.1. Acute Myeloid Leukemia

The various approaches to the induction polychemotherapy of primary acute myeloid leukemia (AML) can achieve complete remissions in 55–70% of adult patients. In more recent studies, the median duration of the first remission is 12–18 months after intensified consolidation therapy, alone or followed by cyclic (prolonged) maintenance therapy. Notwithstanding such remission-maintaining therapeutic modalities, only 10–35% of adults experience disease-free survival within 5 years after attaining complete remission (CR). To date it has not been possible to identify prognostic criteria which are generally valid and also have applicability beyond the various AML studies in adults that might help in reliably estimating the individual risk of relapse at the time of diagnosis or after achievement of remission. The following factors (table 8) therefore still await confirmation of their prognostic value in prospective clinical studies:

Since the mid 1970s, allogeneic BMT has been performed as an intensified postinduction therapy during first CR of AML in patients with HLA-compatible family donors. Meanwhile, an adequate number of reports on long-term observation studies prove without doubt that the risk of relapse can be drastically reduced by this therapeutic measure, compared to chemotherapeutic approaches of remission-maintaining therapy. Although allogeneic marrow transplants during first CR of AML are presently the most effective antileukemic intervention, the indication to perform an allogeneic transplant must take into account that the treatment-related mortality of transplant patients is 10–20% higher than that after chemotherapeutic consolidation or maintenance therapy. Comparisons of the outcome of chemotherapy and of allogeneic BMT in patients with AML in first CR are fundamentally subject to limitations in light of the fact that transplant patients represent a selected population as a consequence of donor availability, patient age, duration of remission at the time of marrow grafting as well as other difficult-to-evaluate criteria. Neither is this fundamental problem of statistical comparison solvable by analytical approaches that try to reduce or compensate for the factors influencing patient selection on the basis of treatment intention (intention-to-treat analysis). A critical note with respect to such analyses is that transplantation results are frequently lopsided. Regardless of the reasons, potential transplant candidates count as BMT failures if they suffer a relapse before a planned transplant, even if the patient himself rejected BMT. Assessment of the efficacy of a treatment modality must be based on patients who were actually treated. A comparison on the intent to treat, however, evaluates fictitious factors, can only reach hypothetical conclusions, and provides no guidelines with regard to the therapeutic decision in individual patients.

For the future, comprehensive prospective studies are necessary which take full account of validated prognostic factors influencing the risk of relapse if a correct assessment of the various therapeutic options available for remission maintenance of AML is to be guaranteed. Table 9 presents a selection of comparative and non-controlled studies on allogeneic BMT in AML performed during first CR.

On the basis of these results it appears justified to conclude that the results of allogeneic BMT in adults with AML in first CR are at least equivalent to those obtained by chemotherapy. According to analyses of major transplantation centers, the 10-year disease-free survival rates are 45–50% for adults transplanted in first CR,

Table 8. Prognostic factors in adult AML

At diagnosis	Favorable	Unfavorable
1. FAB subtype	(M2?), M3, M4Eo	(M5?)
2. Peripheral white blood cells	$<25\times10^9/l$	$\geq25\times10^9/l$
3. CNS- or extramedullary leukemia	not present	present
4. LDH serum activity	<1,000 U/l	≥1,000 U/l
5. Karyotype	t (8; 21) (q22; q22) t (15; 17) (q21; q21) inv(16) (p13; q22)	del5, 5q- del7, 7q- t(9; 22) (q34; q11) inv3 complex anomalies
6. Multidrug resistance (mdr1) gene expression of blasts	not detectable	detectable
7. Dyserythropoiesis or dysmegakaryopoiesis	not present	present
In the course of therapy	**Favorable**	**Unfavorable**
1. Response to induction chemotherapy	CR after 1 to 2 induction courses	no CR after 2 induction courses
2. Minimal residual disease in remission (molecular or immunologic markers)	not detectable	detectable

and the relapse probability is 15–25%. Due to the decrease in lethal transplant-associated complications demonstrable over the past years and the undeniably higher antileukemic efficacy of allogeneic BMT, it can be expected that the long-term results of allogeneic transplant recipients will be superior to those obtained by conventional postinduction chemotherapy. However, the contribution of allogeneic BMT to the overall concept for the treatment of AML is presently rather small. Even at specialized institutions only 60% of those patients in first CR who had an HLA-identical donor actually received a marrow graft because of contraindications or early relapse. With regard to all patients diagnosed with AML, the proportion of patients transplanted in first remission amounted to just around 10%.

Regarding the indication for allogeneic BMT, it can presently be concluded that a transplant should be performed during first CR in those adult patients who have an HLA-genotypically identical sibling or an HLA-phenotypically or HLA-partially matched extended family donor (with a maximum of one serological HLA class I or

Table 9. Results of allogeneic BMT in patients with AML in first CR

Author Study group/center Year of publication	Study design Patient age group, years	Treatment	Follow-up, months	Number of patients	Relapse probability	Event-free survival
Appelbaum Seattle 1988	prospective comparison (intent-to-treat); 17–50 years	patients with donors; BMT performed; consolidation or maintenance	>60–120 >60–120 >60–120	43 33 43	– – –	37 % (10 years) 45 % (10 years) 19 % (10 years)
Büchner German AMLCG 1992	prospective comparison (matched-pair); <60 years	BMT performed; consolidation and maintenance	– –	45 45	– –	65 ± 17 % (5 years) 49 ± 17 % (5 years)
Cassileth ECOG 1992	prospective comparison (intent-to-treat); 41 years	BMT performed; consolidation; maintenance	>12–72 >12–72 >12–72	54 30 21	– – –	42 ± 13 % (6 years) 30 ± 17 % (6 years) 14 ± 15 % (6 years)
Clift Seattle 1987	prospective; uncontrolled; 1–53 years	BMT performed	>12–120	231	25 ± 7 % (5 years)	43 ± 7 % (10 years)
Ferrant Louvain, Brussels 1991	prospective comparison (intent-to-treat); 1–57 years	patients with donors; BMT performed; consolidation	4–48 4–48 4–48	24 20 43	41 ± 12 % (4 years) 33 ± 10 % (4 years) 78 ± 22 % (4 years)	53 ± 19 % (4 years) 64 ± 21 % (4 years) 5 ± 4 % (4 years)
Gratwohl EBMT 1992	prospective comparison (intent-to-treat); 17–57 years	patients with donors; BMT performed; patients without donors	24–48 24–48 24–48	66 48 81	– – –	44 % (4 years) 50 % (4 years) 21 % (4 years)

Author Study group/center Year of publication	Study design Patient age group, years	Treatment	Follow-up, months	Number of patients	Relapse probability	Event-free survival
Horowitz AMLCG/IBMTR 1995	retrospective comparison; 16–50 years	BMT performed;	–	901	–	46 ± 3 % (5 years)
		consolidation and maintenance	–	196	–	34 ± 8 % (5 years)
Reiffers BGMT 1991	prospective comparison (intent-to-treat); 15–55 years	patients with donors;	12–96	60	20 % (3 years)	58 % (3 years)
		patients without donors	12–96	125	52 % (3 years)	35 % (3 years)
Zittoun EORTC-Gimema 1992	prospective comparison; 10–45 years	BMT performed;	–	95		51 ± 10 % (4 years)
		consolidation	–	104		31 ± 11 % (4 years)

II antigen mismatch between donor and recipient). Further prerequisites are that the patient should be less than 55 years of age and have no manifest contraindications like florid or unhealed infections or concomitant diseases that suggest an increased risk of transplant-associated complications. Given these prerequisites, patients with unfavorable prognostic features of de novo AML are urgent candidates for an allogeneic BMT in first CR (fig. 10). The same holds true for patients with secondary AML, developed after successful treatment of a preceding malignant disease or derived from a myelodysplastic syndrome.

Optimally, BMT should be performed within 2–3 months after the patient achieved CR in order to diminish the risk of a relapse before BMT. If a transplant cannot be performed within this time period, consolidation or maintenance chemotherapy should be considered to bridge the waiting time. If the duration of first CR is more than 6 months, the ratio between the chances of cure by chemotherapy alone and the transplantation-associated risks no longer speaks in favor of an indication for allogeneic BMT in first CR.

In children, initial polychemotherapy can induce CR in 70–80%, and the 5-year disease-free survival rates amount to 40–60% after consolidation chemotherapy.

In light of the more favorable results of chemotherapy in children suffering from AML, only those pediatric patients in first CR who have adverse

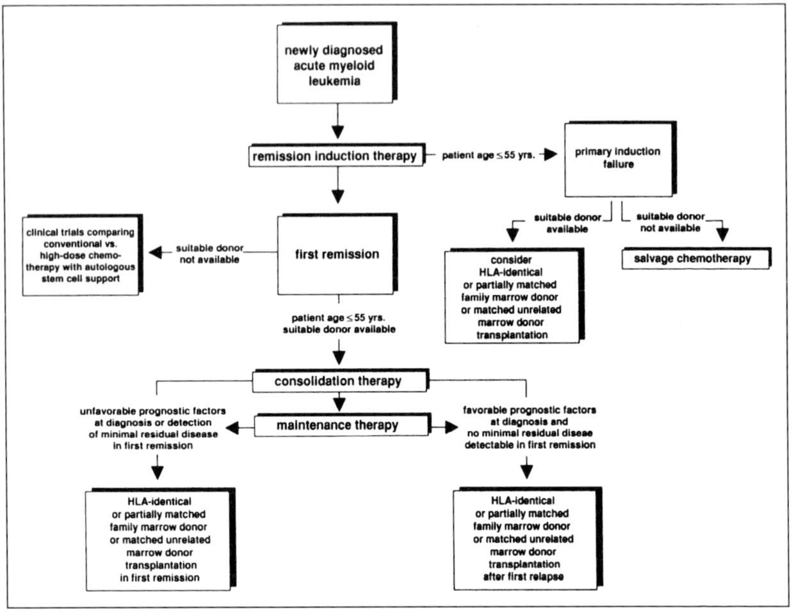

Fig. 10. Decision organigram for the indication of allogeneic BMT in patients with acute myeloid leukemia.

prognostic factors should undergo allogeneic BMT. According to analyses of the Cooperative German Childhood AML Studies, a peripheral blast count of > 100 × 10^9/l and a delayed response to induction therapy were associated with a higher relapse risk.

Since patients with AML who fail induction chemotherapy, and patients in relapse, can be cured hardly by chemotherapeutic measures alone, the following clinical situations pose indisputable and compelling indications for allogeneic BMT in adults as well as children:

1. Failure of induction polychemotherapy with residual disease or with primarily refractory disease;
2. beginning of first relapse;
3. second and consecutive CR.

The higher antileukemic potential of allogeneic BMT is impressively underlined by the fact that BMT was able to induce CRs in around 90% of patients who failed remission induction chemotherapy and that around 20% of these patients were still disease-free after 3 to 5 years. It has furthermore been shown that the 5-year survival rate after allogeneic BMT in incipient first relapse or second CR are identical, i.e., 25–30% (table 10). The therapeutic concept, proposed on the basis of these data, that allogeneic BMT should predominantly be performed in patients who fail primary therapy or after first relapse is hampered by the limited transplantation capacities currently available and by other logistical problems. Therefore this concept is only appropriate in exceptional cases.

In even more advanced stages of disease, around 10% of patients still achieve long-term disease-free survival (table 10).

In patients without histocompatible family marrow donors, allogeneic BMT from a volunteer-unrelated HLA-matched donor is generally not indicated during first remission because of the higher rate of transplant-associated complications. With the exception of unfavorable prognostic disease features, this transplant modality should currently be restricted to patients after the first AML relapse (fig. 10). According to previously published preliminary analyses, only 30–40% of younger transplant patients in first or second CR attained disease-free survival at 2 years. An assessment of the value of allogeneic BMT using unrelated donors within the AML treatment concept is currently not possible due to the low number of treated patients and the short follow-up periods.

New approaches which might contribute to improving the results of allogeneic BMT in AML are currently being examined in the following areas:

1. Enhancement of the antileukemic efficacy with targeted conditioning therapy, e.g., using bone marrow-selective radioimmune conjugates;
2. improvements in the prophylaxis and treatment of acute and chronic graft-versus-host reactions, and development of predictive assays for the early detection of immunological complications;
3. improvements in the prophylaxis and therapy of opportunistic infections;
4. use of hematopoietic growth factors to accelerate hematopoietic reconstitution:
5. detection of minimal residual leukemic cell clones after BMT using molecular genetic assays;
6. immunomodulating interventions in patients with a high risk of relapse or an incipient relapse, e.g., by transfusion of donor blood cells and/or treatment with lymphokines (e.g. interferon-α , interleukin-2).

7.2.2. *Acute Lymphoblastic Leukemia*

According to the results of larger multicenter clinical studies, the initial remission rate in adults with acute lymphoblastic leukemia (ALL) is 65–85%, and around 35% of these patients remain disease-free after consolidation, reinduction and/or mainte-

Table 10. Results of allogeneic BMT in advanced stages of AML

Author Study group/center Year of publication	Disease stage	Number of patients	5-Year relapse probability %	5-Year event-free survival %
Clift Seattle 1987	untreated 1st relapse resistant 1st relapse 2nd remission	54 29 49	36 ± 20 56 ± 26 37 ± 20	30 ± 13 21 ± 14 28 ± 13
Gale IBMTR 1989	2nd remission more advanced stages	229 321	50 70	25 15
Gratwohl EBMT 1992	2nd remission and more advanced stages	149	50	25

nance chemotherapy. The following adverse prognostic factors relating to disease-free survival in adults were identified consistently by most large-scale ALL clinical studies conducted with comparable treatment intensities:

1. Onset of remission > 4–5 weeks after initiation of remission-induction therapy;
2. high initial leukocyte count ($> 30 \times 10^9$/l);
3. higher age (> 50–60 years);
4. chromosomal aberrations: t(9,22) (q34;q11) or bcr-abl-positive ALL; t(4;11)(q21;q23)-positive ALL;
5. immunological markers (B-line ALL).

To date, there is still uncertainty about the prognostic significance of the coexpression of myeloid differentiation surface antigens on ALL blasts which are now more frequently detected due to improvements in immunodiagnostics.

The use of differentiated therapeutic modalities oriented in line with the immunological ALL subtypes has transformed the prognostic significance of the immunological phenotype over the past years. Just a few years ago, T- and B-ALL were classified as prognostically adverse in both children and adults, due to the very low rate of sustained remissions (less than 10%) and the short remission duration. Advances in induction chemotherapy have meanwhile improved the prognosis of these immunologically defined ALL subentities, which is now similar to the prognosis of B-cell precursor (pre-pre-B, common and pre-B) acute leukemias.

Today, special prognostic significance in ALL is given to the cytogenetic detection of the Philadelphia chromosome (Ph') or its molecular genetic equivalent, the bcr-abl hybrid gene. Adult patients with Ph' ALL have a median duration of remission of less than 10 months, and rates of sustained remission are between 0 and 15% in most clinical studies. According to analyses of the Cooperative German Study on Adult ALL, the overall incidence of bcr-abl-positive ALL is 25–30%, and in patients with B-cell precursor ALL it is even 50%. The unfavorable outcomes in adults with ALL compared to those achieved in children must presently be assumed to be partially caused by the fact that the incidence of Ph' ALL increases with age.

The results of allogeneic BMT with histocompatible family donors in patients with ALL must thus be regarded against the background of the biological heterogeneity of the disease and its changing prognostic features. In adults, the published 5-year disease-free survival after allogeneic BMT in first CR ranges between 20 and 60% (table 11). The profound variability of these results might partially be explained by the differing intensities of chemotherapy preceding allogeneic BMT. However, they might additionally reflect the influence of patient selection based on prognostic factors. Generally, the results of allogeneic BMT in adults with ALL in first CR are unsatisfactory. Even in prognostically unfavorable subgroups, retrospective analyses have failed to demonstrate any advantage of allogeneic BMT over consolidation or maintenance chemotherapy in first CR (table 11). The few published retrospective studies conducted on adults with Ph'-(bcr-abl-positive) ALL do indicate, however, that allogeneic BMT in first CR might reduce the relapse risk compared to conventional chemotherapy in spite of the still unacceptably high relapse rates.

Disease-free survival rates between 20 and 40% have been published for allogeneic BMT performed in second CR, and rates of 10 and 30% are being reported in more advanced stages (table 11). These results have led to the consensus that allogeneic BMT is the therapy of choice in adults with histocompatible donors, regardless of prognostic factors after first CR.

According to analyses conducted by the German Pediatric ALL Study Group, allogeneic BMT in patients with histocompatible sibling donors provided a significant advantage with regard to disease-free survival in patients with a bone marrow relapse (regardless of the immunophenotype) within 18 months from diagnosis, or in patients with a relapse of T- or B-ALL (regardless of the relapse localization and duration of first remission), if allogeneic BMT was conducted during second CR. Even when children with very early relapses were included, a disease-free survival rate of around 50% was reported for these patients who otherwise have virtually no chance of cure with conventional chemotherapy.

Allogeneic BMT is basically indicated in adult ALL patients up to the age of 55 years after first relapse, if a histocompatible related or unrelated marrow donor is available and the aforementioned contraindications have been excluded. The Cooperative German Study on Adult ALL is investigating the value of allogeneic BMT in first CR if one of the following adverse prognostic factors is present:

Table 11. Results of allogeneic BMT in patients with ALL

Author Study group/center Year of publication	Disease stage	Number of patients	5-Year relapse probability %	5-Year event-free survival %
Doney Seattle 1991	1st remission 2nd remission 1st or consecutive relapse	41 48 103	50 65 70	21 15 12
Gale IBMTR 1989	1st remission 2nd remission more advanced stages	243 592 281	30 ± 10 60 75	39 ± 10 15 10
Gratwohl EBMT 1988	1st remission 2nd remission and more advanced stages	260 360	25 50	50 30
Horowitz IBMTR/ALL-BMFT 1991	chemotherapy in 1st remission BMT in 1st remission	484 251	59 ± 5 26 ± 7	38 ± 5 44 ± 7
Wingard Baltimore 1990	1st remission 2nd remission 3rd remisson	18 36 16	20 ± 59 26 ± 26 48 ± 32	42 ± 22 43 ± 16 25 ± 23

1. High initial leukocyte counts (> 30 × 10^9/l) in ALL with B-line differentiation (pre-pre-B, common, or B-ALL);
2. Delayed CR (> 4 weeks) regardless of immunological subtype or karyotype;
3. Ph'(bcr-abl)-ALL, t(4;11);
4. Persistent B-ALL after 2–3 blocks of chemotherapy.

Over 90% of children achieve CR through a risk-adapted induction and reinduction chemotherapy, and more than 70% of all afflicted children remain long-term survivors in first CR. The results of conventional chemotherapy, in pediatric patients are thus much more favorable when compared with adults. The indication to perform allogeneic transplants in children during first CR is therefore only accepted if the response to remission induction chemotherapy is delayed, as this is the most important prognostic factor for induction failure as well as for leukemic relapse, and in those few children with Ph' ALL (< 3%). Early relapses within 18 months from diagnosis or relapses of T- or B-ALL are also indications for allogeneic BMT in children with histocompatible family marrow donors. In children with an isolated extramedullary relapse, like testicular or CNS relapse, or late medullary relapses of non-B- or non-T-ALL, the indication for an allogeneic BMT is currently not uniformly accepted.

In addition to the above mentioned therapeutic developments for AML patients in the field of allogeneic BMT, current efforts to improve the unsatisfactory transplant results in ALL patients are especially aimed at reducing the high risk of relapse. A modification of the conditioning treatment in which etoposide, instead of or together with cyclophosphamide, is administered in combination with total-body irradiation (TBI) appears to be particularly promising. Another option represents the combination of high-dose melphalan and TBI. However, a higher antileukemic efficacy of these modifications in comparison to the standard cyclophosphamide and TBI regimen has so far not been demonstrated. The favorable results with hyperfractionated TBI regimens reported by individual centers need also be substantiated by prospective clinical studies.

7.2.3. Chronic Myeloid Leukemia

Although cytoreductive treatment of the chronic phase of chronic myeloid leukemia (CML) using hydroxyurea or busulfan leads to freedom from symptoms in the vast majority of patients, the median survival time is only 40–50 months, and less than 20% of patients treated with these agents survive longer than 5 years. Purified or recombinant human interferon-alpha (IFN-α) alone or in combination with cytostatics (like hydroxyurea or cytosine arabinoside) or other cytokines (like IFN-γ, interleukin-2) is currently being investigated in numerous clinical trials as a new therapeutic option in the chronic phase of CML. Depending on the type of pretreatment, on certain disease and patient characteristics, and in particular on the IFN-α dosage, rates of complete hematologic remissions between 20 and 80% have been reported. An IFN-α-induced suppression of more than 65% of Ph'-positive cells in the bone marrow, which can be demonstrated in 10–20% of IFN-α-treated patients, is associated with a survival probability > 75% after follow-up periods of more than 8 years. However, the published results of molecular genetic analyses demonstrate that even in patients with IFN-α-induced complete cytogenetic remissions the bcr-abl gene rearrangement remains consistently detectable. This suggests that IFN-α treatment is not sufficient to completely suppress or to eliminate the leukemic cell clones, which carry the bcr-abl hybrid gene. Although IFN-α treatment of chronic-phase CML represents a fascinating and effective new therapeutic approach, there is currently no evidence that this approach has curative potential. It ultimately remains to be seen whether the response to IFN-α treatment only contributes to the identification and selection of a patient group, which has a more favorable prognosis per se due to currently undefined tumor biological features of their disease. The extent to which IFN-α therapy improves the prognosis of all treated patients is currently being examined in clinical trials, which compare conventional chemotherapy with IFN-α treatment in the chronic phase of CML.

In around 75% of patients the chronic disease phase is followed by a phase of disease acceleration lasting, on average, 1–1.5 years and ultimately progressing into an acute transformation phase with a predominance of myeloid and lymphatic blasts. In approximately 25% of the patients the terminal acute transformation (also referred to as blastic phase) directly arises from the chronic phase. The prognosis of this terminal disease phase is usually 3–6 months with conventional chemotherapy. In 40–70% of patients with lymphatic blast predominance, combination chemotherapy with vincristine, corticosteroids (and anthracyclines) can induce a second chronic phase which only lasts a few months at the most.

Presently, allogeneic BMT is the only therapeutic modality which leads to long-term hematologic and cytogenetic remissions in most patients with chronic-phase CML. Currently, it remains the sole type of therapy that can permanently eliminate leukemic cells below the sensitivity limits of the molecular genetic methods used to demonstrate the bcr-abl hybrid gene and its products. Given the presently longest follow-up periods for transplant patients of more than 15 years, it appears justified to equate such remissions with a cure of the disease.

The long-term results of allogeneic BMT in the chronic phase published by the larger centers show that disease-free survival reached a stable plateau in 50–60% of patients who received marrow grafts from HLA-identical sibling donors, phenotypically identical or partially HLA-compatible donors (with a maximum of one serologically detectable HLA class I or II antigen mismatch between donor and recipient) from the extended family (table 12). A number of factors were identified which have a crucial effect on the transplant results in patients with chronic-phase CML.

Younger patients who are transplanted within the 1st year of diagnosis have a 3-year disease-free survival rate of 70–90% due to a lower risk of lethal toxic and immunological complications. A longer time interval between diagnosis and allogeneic BMT does not appear to increase the risk of relapse, but rather the transplant-associated mortality which might thus also be negatively influenced by a prolonged cytoreductive chemotherapy of the chronic phase. This especially applies to busulfan pretreatment which is associated with an increased risk of fatal pulmonary complications posttransplant. If the chronic phase lasts more than 1 year, the therapeutic risks of patients older than 30 years are not clearly age-dependent, if other influential factors are considered. A normal or at most slightly enlarged spleen size and absence or only mild marrow fibrosis are considered as prognostically favorable factors with regard to transplant-associated complications, since a pronounced splenomegaly or advanced bone marrow fibrosis may delay hematopoietic reconstitution posttransplant.

Table 12. Results of allogeneic BMT from HLA-identical sibling donors in patients with CML

Author Study group/center Year of publication	Disease stage	Number of patients	Relapse probability	Survival probability
Goldmann/Mc Glave IBMTR 1988/1990	1st chronic phase: T-cell depletion; no T-cell depletion	 87 200	 52 ± 12 % (4 years) 9 ± 4 % (4 years)	 62 ± 11 % (3 years) 58 ± 8 % (3 years)
Gratwohl EBMT 1993	1st chronic phase: T-cell depletion; no T-cell depletion; accelerated phase; blastic phase	 281 666 206 41	 65 ± 10 % (8 years) 21 ± 6 % (8 years) 56 % (5 years) 55 % (2 years)	 21 ± 6 % (8 years)[a] 44 ± 6 % (8 years)[a] 22% (5 years)[a] 17 % (2 years)[a]
Marks London 1992	1st chronic phase: T-cell depletion; MTX/CsA	 51 50	 61 % 6 %	 25 % (5 years)[a] 69 % (5 years)[a]
McGlave IBMTR 1990	1st chronic phase; accelerated phase; blastic phase; 2nd chronic phase	956 392 188 50	13 ± 15 % (4 years) 55 ± 24 % (4 years) 41 ± 39 % (4 years)	53 ± 4 % (6 years) 32 ± 8 % (6 years) 16 ± 6 % (6 years) 25 ± 23 % (3 years)
Thomas Seattle 1989	1st chronic phase	190	24 % (10 years)	65 % (10 years)

[a] Event-free survival.

The gender constellation between bone marrow donor and recipient is relevant to the risk of acute and chronic GvHD. The highest risk is found in male patients with female donors who have been alloimmunized by pregnancies or blood transfusions. This phenomenon points to a possible significance of HY antigens for the development or the clinical severity of GvHD.

The introduction of combined immunoprophylaxis using a short course of methotrexate in combination with ciclosporin led to a significant reduction in the frequency and severity of acute GvHD and consequently to a significant improvement in transplant outcome. This combined immunoprophylaxis has meanwhile become the standard treatment for the prevention of acute GvHD in patients with CML. In contrast, ex vivo depletion of donor T lymphocytes from the graft as prophylaxis of acute GvHD has proven particularly disadvantageous. This technique increases the risk of leukemic recurrence up to 75% as opposed to 15–25% when using unmanipulated marrow grafts. The negative influence of T-cell depletion on the risk of disease recurrence may also be taken as further evidence that immunomechanisms play an important role in the antileukemic effect of allogeneic BMT. In addition, the use of T-cell depletion is associated with an increased risk of primary or secondary graft rejection. The unfavorable transplant results in the chronic phase of CML, published by the European Bone Marrow Transplantation Cooperative Group (EBMTG) on the basis of compiled data from European centers, can at least partially be explained by the fact that the negative influence of T-cell depletion was not always appropriately considered. Another major critical point of such compiled data analyses is that by far not all transplanted patients are reported to the registry, thus placing doubt as to whether these analyses are representative.

In recent years it became apparent that the above-mentioned results of allogeneic BMT in patients with chronic-phase CML who have HLA-compatible intrafamilial donors have been improved by new options for the prevention and treatment of transplant-associated complications. In our patient population (n = 150) the 3-year disease-free survival rate of 50% between 1982 and 1989 has improved to over 85% since 1990. This improvement mainly resulted from a reduction in transplant-related complications. The time period in which the transplant was performed and the immunoprophylaxis of acute GvHD were the two crucial independent prognostic factors for the improvement in disease-free survival.

In the accelerated phase of CML, the disease-free survival probability after allogeneic BMT with an HLA-compatible intrafamilial donor is much poorer than in the chronic phase, due to both an increase in lethal transplant-associated complications and a higher leukemic recurrence rate. Only 10–15% of patients survive, if the transplant is performed during the manifest acute transformation phase. If a second chronic phase by successful chemotherapy of the acute transformation phase can be attained prior to BMT, the disease-free survival rate improves to around 25% (table 12).

Since no other curative therapy besides allogeneic BMT is currently available for CML patients, grafting with marrow from volunteer-unrelated donors is predominantly investigated in this patient group. As a result of the rapidly growing number of registered volunteer donors, a sufficiently histocompatible unrelated donor can now be identified for around 30–40% of patients who have no suitable intrafamilial donor. Should allogeneic BMT with unrelated marrow donors prove its value, the proportion of all CML patients who are potential transplant candidates and might actually receive this type of treatment would rise from 30 to over 60% with the current status of donor registries. In a recent analysis performed by the American National Marrow Donor Program (NMDP), the 2-year disease-free survival estimate was 45% in chronic-phase CML patients who received a bone marrow graft from an unrelated donor within the 1st year from diagnosis and 35% during advanced chronic phase. Lower patient age and complete serological matching of the HLA-A, -B, -DR antigens between donor and recipient represented prognostically favorable features in this analysis. Increased frequencies of severe acute and chronic GvHD, of graft rejections, and of toxic and infectious complications were the leading causes of the inferior transplant results observed among recipients of unrelated donor marrow grafts. According to the NMDP analysis, the 2-year disease-free survival estimate was 20–25% in the accelerated and the 2nd chronic phase, while no patient survived who received a transplant during manifest blastic phase.

The previously published data on allogeneic BMT with marrow from unrelated donors must be assessed with caution, considering that the patients treated were selected primarily on the basis of poor prognostic factors. Recent developments in histocompatibility testing, the rapidly growing number of available donors, and advances in the prophylaxis and therapy of transplant-associated complications justify the expectation that the results of unrelated marrow donor transplants will be improved in the near future.

Despite the promising results of IFN-α therapy, allogeneic BMT with histocompatible intrafamilial donors is unreservedly indicated at the earliest possible time in patients with newly diagnosed CML up to the age of 50 to 55 years (fig. 11). In patients up to the age of 60 years who generally qualify for allogeneic BMT, a 12-month treatment course with IFN-α should be attempted. In those patients who achieve a partial or complete cytogenetic response, IFN-α therapy should be continued until loss of efficacy. If there is no response within 12 months (Ph'-positive bone marrow cells > 50%), allogeneic BMT should be ventured in this age group. If cytoreductive therapy is necessary in newly diagnosed CML to bridge the time up to a planned BMT, it should be performed with hydroxyurea, since busulfan (and possibly IFN-α) raises the risk of transplant-associated complications. In patients with a longer course of the chronic phase, which is successfully controlled by IFN-α (Ph'-positive bone marrow cells < 35%), the indication for an allogeneic BMT arises only at the time of subsiding IFN-α efficacy and disease progression. All other patients on conventional cytoreductive therapy of the chronic phase who have a suitable intrafamilial marrow donor should undergo transplantation as early as possible.

Allogeneic BMT from a histocompatible unrelated marrow donor is indicated in chronic-phase CML patients without a suitable intrafamilial donor up to the age of 50 years, if they are primary nonresponders to a 12-month IFN-α treatment course or if they do no longer respond after more than 12 months of IFN-α treatment. Furthermore, all patients in advanced chronic phase under conventional cytoreductive therapy and particularly after the first signs of disease progression should be grafted with marrow from unrelated donors, if suitable intrafamilial donors are not available. As disease-specific contraindications, massive, untreatable splenomegaly and/or advanced bone marrow fibrosis may be considered. Both the accelerated phase and the second chronic phase of CML present compelling indications for allogeneic BMT with either histocompatible intrafamilial or unrelated donors. In manifest blast crisis, BMT with an unrelated donor is, in turn, only justifiable if the

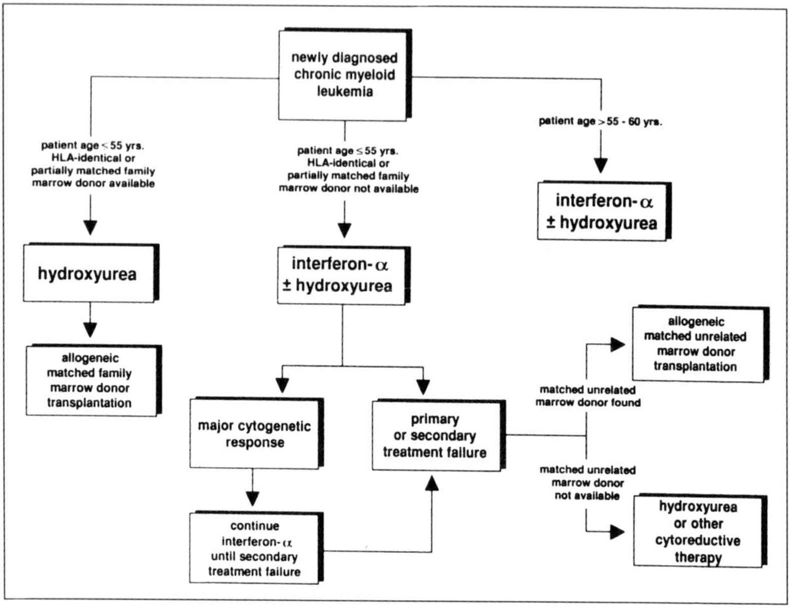

Fig. 11. Decision organigram for the indication of allogeneic BMT in patients with chronic myeloid leukemia.

tumor mass is controlled, i.e., if there is less than 50% blast infiltration of the bone marrow and no massive splenomegaly. Furthermore, the patient's general status during the time required to organize the transplant should, as far as predictable, remain stable and not substantially reduced.

Particular interest is currently directed towards the clinical significance of the detection of minimal residual disease markers of CML posttransplant. The gene sequence-specific amplification of the bcr-abl gene transcript as a molecular genetic equivalent to the Ph' chromosome using the polymerase chain reaction (PCR) allows the detection of one malignant among 10^5 to 10^6 normal cells. First results of sequential studies on the bcr-abl status suggest that an intermittent, but especially a persistent PCR positivity more than 1 year posttransplant indicates a greatly increased risk of disease recurrence. On the other hand, positive results within the first months after BMT appear to be of little predictive value for disease recurrence. These studies might form the basis for prophylactic interventions aimed at reducing the risk of leukemic relapse. In this context, some interesting ongoing investigations have shown that in a high percentage of patients with cytogenetic or hematologic relapse after allogeneic BMT, complete and long-term Ph' negativity can be induced by transfusions of peripheral blood cells from the bone marrow donor. Although the cellular mechanisms of the antileukemic effect of "donor buffy coat" transfusions have not yet been elucidated, it can be assumed that this phenomenon is caused by donor-alloreactive T lymphocytes in terms of the graft-versus-leukemia (GvL) effect. Not all patients who respond to this treatment develop transfusion-associated GvHD, opening up the possibility that GvHD and the GLV effect are attributable to clinically separate immunomechanisms. Furthermore, it is currently being tested whether IFN-α therapy during the early posttransplant course can reduce the frequency of relapse in patients with an increased relapse risk.

The majority of relapses observed after allogeneic BMT occurs within the first 2 years posttransplant. With rare exceptions, the disease stage of the relapse corresponds to the stage of CML that existed at the time of transplantation. It must also be stressed that even hematologic relapses after allogeneic BMT can be treated with curative intent. In younger patients a second transplant appears promising if the time interval between the first BMT and relapse is longer than 1 year. According to data of the EBMTG and of individual centers, long-term disease-free survival in the range of 20% can be attained by a 2nd BMT with an HLA-identical intrafamilial donor. Depending on the disease activity, different modalities may be used for the treatment of CML relapse posttransplant. If repeated cytogenetic analyses reveal an increasing number of Ph'-positive bone marrow cells more than 6 months after BMT without an overt hematologic relapse, immunosuppressive prophylaxis or therapy of chronic GvHD should be reduced or stopped, since sustained Ph' negativity can occasionally be achieved by this measure alone. Based on the published promising results, donor buffy-coat transfusions may primarily be attempted in case of an incipient hematologic relapse. In nonresponding patients, IFN-α therapy should be initiated, since a recent analysis suggested that IFN-α is more effective than conventional cytoreductive agents for the treatment of posttransplant CML relapse. In patients with partial or complete cytogenetic responses, this therapy should be continued until loss of efficacy. In younger patients with late relapses (> 1 year post-BMT), the question of a second marrow graft should be alternatively considered.

7.2.4. Myelodysplastic Syndromes

Allogeneic BMT currently represents the sole curative therapeutic approach to the heterogenic disease group of primary and secondary myelodysplastic syndromes (MDS). The median age of patients afflicted by these diseases is in the 7th decade of life, and disease manifestations in childhood or adolescence are correspondingly rare. In the light of this age distribution, only the small fraction of patients under the age of 50–55 years with histocompatible donors can be treated by an allogeneic transplant. Similar to the results of polychemotherapy in MDS during leukemic transformation, the results of allogeneic BMT are also less favorable than those reported for transplants in patients with primary AML. In an analysis of European transplant centers, the 5-year disease-free survival estimate was around 25% for all patients with MDS or secondary leukemias after allogeneic BMT with a histocompatible intrafamilial marrow donor. In subgroups of younger patients who achieved CRs before BMT or with early disease stages, a 5-year disease-free survival estimate of 40–50% has been reported. Initial experience using allogeneic BMT with unrelated marrow donors gained by the NMDP in MDS patients produced a 2-year disease-free survival estimate of only 15–20%, although these results can partially be explained by the selection of patients with poor prognostic factors.

A decision as to the indication for allogeneic BMT in patients with MDS must consider the prognosis in relation to the morphological subgroup, age, and other prognostic factors (cytogenetics, blast infiltration of the bone marrow, severity of granulocytopenia and/or thrombocytopenia, lactate dehydrogenase elevation, DNA aneuploidy, etc.). One has to be aware, however, that the aforementioned factors are only of limited predictive value in individual cases. In morphological subgroups that do not show detectable malignant transformation (refractory anemia or refractory anemia with ring sideroblasts) and whose survival estimate with supportive therapy alone ranges between 20 and 80 months, the indication to perform an allogeneic BMT may depend on the judgement of the vital danger related to the degree of granulocytopenia and/or thrombocytopenia. In cases of doubt, monitoring the clinical course of the tendency to infections or hemorrhages can reinforce the decision. Allogeneic BMT is generally indicated in all morphological subgroups with clonal malignant transformation (refractory anemia with blast excess, refractory anemia with blast excess in transformation, chronic myelomonocytic leukemia). In an individual patient, an assessment should be made as to whether remission or reduction of the malignant clone induced by polychemotherapy may be advantageous prior to BMT. However, the benefits and risks of this prior therapeutic intervention should be carefully weighted in the light of the high rate of severe and life-threatening complications of conventional polychemotherapy in MDS patients. Since the most favorable results with allogeneic BMT have been achieved in younger patients without malignant transformation of MDS, future studies should clarify whether it is justified to take a wait-and-see stance until malignant transformation.

A particular problem is posed by patients who have developed MDS as a secondary disease after successful chemotherapy and/or radiotherapy of a prior malignant disease. If it can be assumed that the primary malignant disease has been treated curatively, the indication for an allogeneic BMT should be rendered in view of the extremely poor prognosis of secondary forms of MDS. A concomitant pronounced marrow fibrosis or massive splenomegaly, which is more frequently observed among patients with chronic myelomonocytic leukemia, may present major obstacles for a successful allogeneic BMT.

7.3. Severe Combined Immunodeficiency

Severe combined immunodeficiency (SCID) is characterized by congenital defects in the humoral as well as the cellular immune system. The syndrome often manifests in the first months of life and is usually fatal within the 1st year, due to recurring infections. It includes a variety of heterogeneous diseases in which the B-cell system or the T-cell system of the lymphopoiesis is impaired to varying degrees. Defects of the complement system or the monocyte-macrophage system can also be present. Combinations with other somatic disorders are not uncommon. Inheritance and pathogenesis of SCID vary. As a possible cause of SCID, defects in the hematopoietic stem cells are under discussion. The number of T and B lymphocytes is extremely reduced, and agammaglobulinemia with defective or complete absence of antibody production is frequently found. Autosomal recessive as well as X-chromosomal recessive heredity are both possible.

For 20 years, allogeneic BMT has been the treatment of choice for SCID patients. When an HLA-genotypically identical donor is available, over half of the patients achieve reconstitution of the immune system and long-term survival. In the majority of patients, the graft lymphopoiesis is accepted without any conditioning pretreatment. Sometimes, however, only the donor T-cell lymphopoiesis engrafts while B cells remain of recipient type and functionally impaired. The recipient's non-lymphatic hematopoiesis is generally normal.

Since most patients do not have an HLA-identical donor available, transplantation using marrow of haploidentical family members has been performed with increasing frequency in recent years. The graft is first treated in vitro to remove the T cells and reduce the risk of acute GvHD. The preferred method of T-cell depletion ex vivo consists of incubation of the marrow graft with T-cell-specific cytotoxic antibodies followed by complement lysis. This is followed by physical separation techniques using immunomagnetic antibody-coated beads or rosette formation after lectin agglutination. As mentioned previously, transplantation of leukemia patients with T-cell-depleted marrow leads to a significant proportion of graft rejections, even though the incidence of GvHD can be reliably reduced. In patients with congenital SCID, transplantation of T-cell-depleted marrow from haploidentical donors results in donor-type T-cell reconstitution in the majority of cases without conditioning pretreatment. The development of B-cell functions, on the other hand, is seldom observed. As a rule, donor B cells do not engraft and the patient's own B cells, which are sometimes already present, do not take on any specific functions in spite of the T-cell reconstitution. The results obtained with haploidentical T-cell-depleted grafts in an increasing number of SCID patients are promising, even when retransplantation or cytoreductive pretreatment is sometimes necessary. Transplantations with unrelated donors have been attempted in a few SCID patients, but are still of experimental nature.

7.4. Rare and Experimental Indications

Allogeneic BMT is an established therapy for SCID. Wiscott-Aldrich syndrome, which is characterized by functional disorders of lymphocytes and platelets, can also be cured with allogeneic BMT. Other congenital disorders of the hematopoietic system which can successfully be treated with allogeneic transplantation include agranulocytosis, chronic granulomatosis, Chediak-Higashi syndrome, juvenile osteopetrosis, Blackfan-Diamond anemia, Fanconi's anemia, sickle-cell anemia and thalassemia major.

In thalassemia major, most patients can achieve long-term survival when the decision for transplantation is made early in the disease course. In diseases spanning several years, the success of transplantation may be endangered by iron overload, chronic hepatitis, and periportal fibrosclerosis of the liver.

The transplantation group in Pesaro (Italy) reported on over 156 children with thalassemia major who received allogeneic BMT after conditioning with busulfan and cyclophosphamide. The average age of patients was 8 years. 87% of these children survived relapse-free. The maximum observation time was 1,500 days. The relapse rate was given as 7%.

Since the monocyte-macrophage system is populated by donor cells after allogeneic BMT, it seems reasonable to investigate the therapeutic value of congenital lysosomal thesaurismoses such as Hurler's syndrome, Sanfilippo's syndrome and metachromatic leukodystrophy. Data on over 100 children grafted for these diseases have been collected. In some cases, improvement in growth, physical development, and in cerebral functions have been reported.

Whether solid tumors can be successfully treated with allogeneic BMT has received little attention up to now. Current major clinical trials focus on high-dose therapy with autologous stem cell support in patients with advanced breast cancer, germ-cell malignancies, neuroblastoma, and soft-tissue sarcomas, like Ewing's sarcoma as well as osteosarcoma.

8. Complications of Bone Marrow Transplantation

Complications associated with allogeneic BMT result primarily from the adverse effects of the myeloablative conditioning therapy, immunological problems due to genetic disparities between donor and recipient, and the biological behavior of the underlying disease after transplantation (table 13).

8.1. Early Toxicity

Immediately following TBI, dizziness, nausea and vomiting develop in varying intensities. Parotid swellings and erythrodermia are also typical and can persist for a couple of days. Unfractionated TBI is often followed by elevated body temperatures, tachycardia, and chills as a result of cell destruction and lymphokine release. These immediate adverse effects of the conditioning regimen are greatly reduced when TBI is given in fractionated doses over a period of several days. The cumulative toxicity of TBI, chemotherapy, and of immunoprophylaxis with methotrexate leads to lesions of the mucous membranes of the respiratory and gastrointestinal tracts. These usually appear as erosive and/or ulcerative changes and are accompanied by substantial dysphagia and watery diarrhea. In extreme cases the damage to the oropharyngeal mucosa is so pronounced that the upper airways are obstructed by mucous membranes. Increased secretion and bleeding can make intubation necessary to overcome the danger of aspiration.

In addition to the emetogenic effects of high-dose cyclophosphamide as the most widely used chemotherapeutic agent prior to allogeneic BMT, its cardiotoxic side effects, particularly in patients with preexisting cardiac damage or disease, have to be considered. Further, the urinary bladder mucosa may be damaged by toxic metabolites of cyclophosphamide, but this adverse effect can be avoided by forced diuresis, urine alkalization, and the application of mesna as a specific antidote. Hair loss, which typically occurs during the first 2 posttransplant weeks, is completely reversible within 6 months after transplantation. The prophylactic use of ciclosporin A may be accompanied by systemic hypertension, disturbances in kidney and liver functions, and adverse effects on the central nervous system. In most instances these early adverse ciclosporin A effects are reversible and can be ameliorated by dosage adjustments according to the monitoring of blood levels of ciclosporin A.

Table 13. Major problems of allogeneic BMT

1. Early toxicity of radiochemotherapy
Reversible adverse effects
Nausea and vomiting
Mucositis
Diarrhea
Hemorrhagic cystitis
Marrow aplasia (infections, bleeding complications)
Alopecia
Parotitis
Life threatening adverse effects
Interstitial pneumonia
Hepatic veno-occlusive disease
Congestive cardiomyopathy
2. Late toxicity of radiochemotherapy
Gonadal insufficiency (sterility)
Growth disturbances in children
Cataracts
Secondary malignancies
3. Graft rejection
4. GvHD
5. Leukemic relapse

Increased capillary permeability in the early posttransplant period with a generalized tendency to edema, weight gain and, most seriously, interstitial edema of the lungs (referred to as capillary leak syndrome) has been first reported in patients receiving ciclosporin-A-containing immunoprophylactic regimens who have been transplanted with marrow from partial HLA-compatible family donors. This clinical syndrome has now to be regarded primarily as a consequence of direct toxic effects of high-dose therapy on the endothelium of small blood vessels, which is further modulated by the activation of different pathways of acute inflammation. Fluid retention caused by this syndrome may be further enhanced by fluid overload due to parental nutrition or treatment with systemic antibiotics containing high sodium concentrations.

In about 10–20% of patients, acute liver dysfunction manifests typically within the first 2 posttransplant weeks and is caused by subintimal edema in the terminal liver veins with consecutive intraluminar collagen accumulation. This is clinically characterized by a sudden painful enlargement of the liver, an increase in body weight due to ascites and generalized edema, signs of portal hypertension and cholestatic jaundice. This liver disorder, referred to as hepatic veno-occlusive disease (VOD), has to be regarded as a consequence of cumulative liver toxicity of high-dose therapy, which is modulated by pre- and posttransplant toxic as well as infectious risk factors. Most centers are now using prophylactic heparin for the prevention of hepatic VOD. Therapy for hepatic VOD is limited to symptomatic measures such as avoiding potentially hepatotoxic agents, restricting fluid intake, albumin substitution, and careful use of aldosterone-antagonistic diuretics. The successful therapeutic use of synthetic prostaglandins or activators of fibrinolysis for the treatment of VOD has been repeatedly reported.

As a consequence of the toxicity on hematopoietic tissues, the first 3–4 weeks after transplantation are characterized by symptoms related to lymphohematopoietic insufficiency, which is predominantly characterized by thrombocytopenic bleeding tendency and profound susceptibility to infections. To compensate for reduced food intake, malabsorption of nutrients and the resulting catabolism, parenteral hyperalimentation is generally necessary in the first weeks after transplantation.

8.2. Late Toxicity

Organ function impairments which manifest later than 100 days after transplantation can seldom be unequivocally identified as late toxic sequelae of the pretransplant conditioning regimen, because a distinction between the effects of immunologic or infectious complications and other consequences of therapy is often impossible. One well-known late complication of radiation exposure is cataracts. Since shielding of the eyes is not possible during TBI due to possible leukemic involvement, it is inevitable that some patients will develop cataracts. The introduction of fractionated TBI has reduced the incidence from 75–80% in patients receiving single-dose exposure to about 20% within the first 6 years after transplantation. The relationship between radiation dose, dose rates and fractionation schedules of TBI and the risk of cataracts is still unclear. If long-term treatment with corticosteroids is necessary because of chronic GvHD, cataracts occur more frequently, earlier, and also in patients treated exclusively with cyclophosphamide prior to transplantation.

Pulmonary function analyses have revealed asymptomatic disturbances of gas exchange in most patients after TBI. In a large study 20% of patients showed minor restrictive ventilation dysfunctions, which regressed with increasing time after transplantation. In association with chronic GvHD, however, obstructive ventilation disorders can develop, which take on the clinical and histological characteristics of obliterative bronchiolitis. Under discussion as possible causes for obstructive airway diseases after transplantation are a disturbed bronchial secretion, recurring bronchopulmonary infections, and immune mechanisms.

The combination of TBI and high-dose cyclophosphamide leads to severe disorders in endocrine and reproductive gonadal functions. Female patients develop ovarian insufficiency which is nearly always irreversible and in about 50% of women is accompanied by menopausal symptoms. All female patients will require hormone substitution on a regular basis for the rest of their lives to prevent secondary complications which result from the combined deficiency of estrogens and gestagens. Male patients develop azoospermia which, with rare exceptions, is also irreversible. The gonadal production of testosterone in male patients, however, is usually normal, and hormone substitution is indicated only in cases of proven testosterone deficiency.

In patients with SAA, who were exclusively pretreated with cyclophosphamide, the hormonal situation appears similar to conventional chemotherapy with alkylating agents in that the gonadal function after therapy depends on the patient's age and the duration and dosage of chemotherapy. Younger women often develop a normal menstruation cycle, and men usually have normal hormone production and spermatogenesis. After high-dose cyclophosphamide conditioning, numerous pregnancies and deliveries of healthy children have been reported. More recently, even a few female patients who had been pretreated by TBI have had pregnancies, which resulted in the birth of healthy children.

In prepubescent children, combined radiochemotherapy results in the absence or delay in the development of secondary sex characteristics and absence of sexual functions. Particular note should be given to the fact that the majority of total-body-irradiated children develop growth disorders. In about one third of these children a lack of growth hormone and adrenal steroids can be detected, which must be corrected using substitution therapy targeted to initiate growth and development of secondary sex characteristics. Children who received only high-dose cyclophosphamide, by comparison, generally grow and develop normally.

Beside the abnormal gonadal endocrine functions, about half of patients after TBI show a temporary malfunction of the thyroid gland on a subclinical level, which can be detected by an increase in thyroid-stimulating hormone levels.

On the basis of data from animal experiments it must be assumed that radiochemotherapeutic conditioning increases the risk of developing secondary malignancies. Among marrow transplantation patients there are increasing numbers of reports on secondary malignancies that may have been caused by the radiochemotherapeutic pretreatment and the posttransplant immunosuppression. Within the first 2 years, lymphoproliferative disorders appear to be particularly prevalent. These lymphomas predominantly originate in the B-cell system, and there is evidence for a connection to Epstein-Barr virus infections. The extent to which posttransplant immunosuppression leads to T-cell dysfunction and uncontrolled B-cell proliferation is still open. In this context it appears significant that Epstein-Barr virus associated-lymphoproliferative diseases are preferably observed among patients after T-cell depletion or in vivo administration of T-cell-specific monoclonal antibodies or ATG. The relatively small number of patients under long-term observation after combined radiochemotherapy followed by marrow transplantation does not permit any definitive conclusions regarding the risk of secondary malignancies. Currently there is growing evidence, however, that long-term survivors carry an increased risk to develop solid tumors. Especially, epithelial cancers of the oral mucous membranes seem to be more frequent among these patients.

8.3. Infectious Complications

Extreme susceptibility to infections in the early phase after BMT is attributable to several factors: In addition to toxic lesions of the skin and the mucous membranes of varying intensity, which permit exogenous germ invasion, cellular lymphohematopoietic insufficiency, accompanied by profound pancytopenia and dysfunction of the humoral immunity, leads to a pronounced susceptibility to a wide spectrum of pathogens. The necessity of using permanent central venous catheters, the high demand for blood component substitution, and the immunosuppressive treatment following transplantation also contribute to a predisposition to infections. During the first 3 to 4 weeks after transplantation, most patients develop fever and in 30–40% of patients, blood cultures show bacterial pathogens during this period of extreme granulocytopenia in spite of the preventive measures described. In recent years, gram-positive bacteria, like coagulase-negative Staphylococci and Corynebacteria, are the most common causes of febrile episodes in granulocytopenic transplant patients. Despite the frequent detection of pathogens in blood cultures, bacterial organ infections in the early posttransplant phase are not common.

Although mycotic colonization of the gastrointestinal mucous membranes is frequently observed, systemic or organ infections from Candida or Aspergillus are uncommon in the early posttransplant period.

As a consequence of an endogenous reactivation, about 50% of patients show herpes simplex virus (HSV) excretion in the oral cavity within the first posttransplant weeks. The most frequent clinical manifestation of HSV reactivation is an often severe and painful gingivostomatitis. Genital, intestinal or generalized manifestations of HSV infections are rarely observed.

Thanks to gnotobiotic surveillance, infection-preventive measures and the timely use of systemic broad-spectrum antibiotics, antimycotics and acyclovir, life-threatening infections during the phase of severe granulocytopenia have become rare, and the mortality from these early infectious complications is now in the range of 5%. After peripheral blood neutrophil counts have increased to over $0.5–1 \times 10^9/l$, fever usually disappears and bacterial or mycotic infections in patients not developing acute GvHD are the exception.

Over a period of several months, all patients exhibit a pronounced susceptibility to viral infections as a result of the persisting deficiency of the specific cellular and humoral immune system. These infections are most frequently caused by DNA viruses and among these, herpes viruses have the highest prevalence. About 50% of seropositive patients develop localized varicella-zoster virus (VSV) infections, while generalized infections or organ manifestations from VSV are rarely observed, if systemic acyclovir therapy is timely instituted. Exogenous infections or the reactivation of latent infections with Epstein-Barr virus appear to progress without symptoms in most cases. In contrast, gastroenteritis caused by enteropathogenic viruses, such as adenovirus, rotavirus or coxsackievirus, are occasionally seen and usually manifest as nonspecific gastroenteritis. Other opportunistic pathogens, like *Toxoplasma gondii*, Mycobacteria, Cryptococci, Legionellae, Mycoplasma, Chlamydia and others can cause local or disseminated infections predominantly in patients suffering from acute or chronic GvHD. Since the introduction of oral trimethoprim-sulfamethoxazol prophylaxis, *Pneumocystis carinii* pneumonia has become a rare infectious complication in transplant recipients.

Due to their high prevalence and their major impact on morbidity and mortality of marrow transplant recipients, infections with cytomegalovirus (CMV) are of particular importance. Latent CMV infections can progress with largely varying severity. The spectrum of CMV disease includes oligosymptomatic viremia, enteritis, esophagitis, hepatitis, persistent fever, encephalitis (possibly combined with retinochorioiditis), impairment of bone marrow function, and interstitial pneumonia. In seropositive patients, the vast majority of these symptomatic infections results from reactivation of latent infections. In seronegative patients, blood products from CMV antibody-positive blood or bone marrow donors are the major source of virus transmission. Thus, the most effective measure to prevent CMV disease in seronegative patients is the omission of CMV transmission, whenever possible. In seronegative patients grafted with marrow from a seronegative donor, exogenous infections can be almost completely prevented by using blood cell substitution from CMV antibody-negative blood donors. The efficacy of passive immunoprophylaxis using repeated intravenous immunoglobulin preparations with high concentrations of CMV-specific antibodies (hyperimmunoglobulins) cannot be regarded as established at present. Several prospective studies investigating the efficacy of passive immunoprophylaxis using different preparations of hyperimmunoglobulins in BMT patients reported results ranging from effective suppression of CMV disease including CMV interstitial pneumonia to a complete failure in preventing CMV disease. In seropositive patients, there is no evidence at all to support that passive immunization is effective in reducing the risk of CMV disease.

A controlled study of high-dose prophylactic acyclovir in seropositive transplant patients revealed a significant reduction in the incidences of CMV pneumonia and of reactivation of latent infections. Currently, clinical trials focus on the efficacy of the antiviral agents ganciclovir or foscavir, both of which show greater in vitro activity against CMV compared to acyclovir, to prevent CMV disease in BMT recipients. The first two of these prospective randomized trials, in which the application of ganciclovir was investigated on the basis of a positive rapid virus culture assay ("preemptive therapy"), revealed a significantly reduced incidence of CMV disease. Two other studies investigating the prophylactic use of ganciclovir during the early posttransplant period independent from the proof of viral replication demonstrated a significant reduction in CMV infections and disease. As a consequence of the marrow toxicity of ganciclovir, a high incidence of neutropenia (30–50%) was observed in these four studies. Further, a significantly increased risk of bacterial infections during ganciclovir-induced neutropenia was described in one of these studies. A positive influence on transplant-related mortality during the first 100 posttransplant days was noted in one of the studies, which investigated preemptive ganciclovir therapy. The currently available results support the use of ganciclovir during the early posttransplant period only in those patients who have virologic evidence for CMV replication as detected by rapid culture techniques or, more recently, by CMV antigenemia assay.

For the treatment of manifest CMV disease and especially CMV interstitial pneumonia, the combination of ganciclovir and hyperimmunoglobulin currently appears to have the highest efficacy. Using this therapy, still more than 50% of affected patients will die from this complication, and recurrence of CMV interstitial pneumonia in successfully treated patients remains common. Another therapeutic option for the treatment of CMV disease is the combination of foscarnet and ganciclovir, although controlled studies investigating this option in comparison to ganciclovir alone or in combination with hyperimmunoglobulins have so far not been reported.

As a consequence of the persisting humoral and cellular immunodeficiency, late infectious complications are more frequently observed among patients with primary or secondary chronic GvHD, whereas patients with undisturbed lymphohematopoietic reconstitution seldom develop infections later than 4 to 6 months after transplantation. Patients with chronic GvHD generally tend toward recurring infections of the nasal sinuses and the respiratory tract as well as toward bacteremia. These are most frequently caused by gram-positive cocci and among these, *Staphylococcus aureus* and Pneumococci are predominant. Disturbance of the mucous membranes that results from xerostomia, associated with chronic GvHD, additionally leads to an increased susceptibility to mycotic colonization of the upper gastrointestinal and respiratory tracts as well as to recurring HSV stomatitis. Additional explanations for the increased incidence of airway infections in patients with chronic GvHD include impairment of the chemotactic functions of granulocytes and monocytes, a reduced topical secretion of IgA, and impaired production of specific antibodies for Pneumococci-polysaccharide. It is further assumed that functional hyposplenism contributes to persistent susceptibility to infections.

Patients who have been grafted with marrow from HLA-partially compatible family donors appear to have a higher rate of early and late infectious complications as opposed to patients who received their transplant from an HLA-genotypically identical sibling donor. This adverse effect of HLA mismatching seems to depend not only on the increased incidence of acute or chronic GvHD.

8.4. Interstitial Pneumonia

Interstitial pneumonia (IP) develops in 10–40% of patients after allogeneic BMT. In previous years this complication had a fatal course in the majority of affected patients and was thus one of the leading causes of transplant-associated mortality. The pathogenic mechanisms of IP after BMT are currently unexplained. One decisive factor of this pulmonary complication is the pretransplant conditioning regimen. About 10% of patients with aplastic anemia, who were exclusively conditioned with cyclophosphamide, developed IP. In contrast, the frequency among leukemia patients who received TBI was reported to be 30–40%. A retrospective multivariate analysis of the IBMTR in 932 leukemia patients whose conditioning included TBI identified the following factors as having a significant impact on the risk of IP:

1. The risk was 2.3-fold increased in patients who received methotrexate as prophylaxis for acute GvHD compared to patients with ciclosporin prophylaxis.
2. In patients with acute GvHD of grades II-IV, the risk was 1.9-fold higher as opposed to patients with grades 0-I acute GvHD.
3. Patients older than 21 years had a 2.1-fold higher risk compared with younger patients.
4. The risk increased by a factor of 1.6 when the time between diagnosis and transplantation was more than 6 months, as compared to a shorter interval.
5. A reduced performance status at the time of transplantation was associated with a 2.1-fold higher risk.
6. TBI with a dose rate over 4 cGy/min increased the risk among patients treated with methotrexate prophylaxis by a factor of 3.2, compared to patients irradiated with lower dose rates. In patients receiving ciclosporin prophylaxis, dose rates between 2 and 108 cGy/min had no impact on the probability of IP.

In a comparable IBMTR analysis of 439 patients with aplastic anemia, the above mentioned risk factors 1 to 3 had a similar significance on the risk of IP. It was further demonstrated by this analysis that combined radiochemotherapeutic conditioning regimens increased this risk of IP compared to chemotherapy alone: The respective figures for TBI-containing regimens, total lymphatic irradiation or thoracoabdominal irradiation, and sole chemotherapy were 32, 17, and 8%.

A phenomenologic classification discriminating between infectious and idiopathic IPs, in which a causative agent cannot be identified, is generally used in the literature. The proportion of infectious IPs is presumed to be in the range of 50%. This estimate, however, may be too low if the technical difficulties in obtaining sufficient specimens for diagnosis and the logistical problems of isolating and identifying causative pathogens are taken into consideration. In 80–90% of infectious IPs, CMV has been identified as the underlying pathogen. Other less common pathogens include herpes simplex or varicella-zoster virus, adenovirus, Candida, Aspergillus or *Pneumocystis carinii*. Regardless of the CMV serologic status prior to transplantation, approximately 30-40% of patients with CMV disease previously developed CMV IP posttransplant.

Decisive pathogenic factors in idiopathic IP include toxic damage to the lung tissue resulting from chemotherapeutic treatment of the primary disease, the radiochemotherapeutic conditioning, and the immunosuppressive therapy after transplantation. The part played by each individual factor in the pathogenic sequence leading to IP cannot be more closely defined yet. Although TBI per se is without doubt a determining factor in IP, the type of application – apart from the previously described effect of the dose rate – appears to play a subordinate role. In the analyses cited, neither varying the fractionation, nor an average lung dose between 5.6 and 12.8 Gy had an effect on the risk of idiopathic IP. To what extent a decrease of the effective radiation dose to the lungs to 8–10 Gy reduces pulmonary toxicity is at present unknown.

It is interesting to note that, despite a comparable intensity of the pretreatment, CMV IP occurs less frequently after syngeneic or autologous BMT. To what extent this reduced incidence reflects the impact of immunologic factors or immunosuppressive treatment following allogeneic transplantation is unclear. The pathogenesis of CMV infections depends to a great extent on the humoral, and particularly on the cellular, immunity of the infected organism. It can be therefore assumed that the immunosuppressive therapy after transplantation has a negative impact on the course of such infections, and thus predisposes to the patients' CMV IP. The pronounced impairments of specific humoral and cellular immunity during acute or chronic GvHD could similarly favor development of this complication. All in all, the multitude of known factors serves to underline the complexity of the pathogenesis of posttransplant IP.

IPs usually develop between 30 and 100 days after transplantation. This suggests that effector cells of the graft, or mediators produced by these cells, contribute to the pathologic reaction of the lung tissue. About 80% of IPs occur during this period, and about 90% are observed within the first 6 months after transplantation. After that, this lung complication is only observed in isolated cases and more or less exclusively in patients with chronic GvHD.

Predominant clinical symptoms of IP are a creeping or fulminant respiratory insufficiency with progressive dyspnea and tachypnea, unproductive cough and cyanosis, occasionally accompanied by fever. Blood gas analysis regularly shows hypoxemia, which initially may be accompanied by normocapnia or hypocapnia. Pulmonary function tests reveal a constellation of a restrictive ventilation disorder with reduced lung volumes, reduced compliance, and decreased diffusion capacity. In thoracic X-rays fine reticular bilateral interstitial markings predominate. Initially, these are often more pronounced in the basal and hilus regions of the lung. Superinfections, however, can also cause confluent infiltrates. As the disease progresses, these changes gradually diffuse throughout the lungs. In X-rays they show up as a milky-glass-like opaqueness of the infiltrated areas (fig. 12).

Histologic changes in the acute stage include diffuse alveolitis with interstitial edema, cellular infiltrations of the interstitium as well as alveolar exudates and, in advanced stages, fibrosis of the lung interstitium. Figure 13 shows the histologic changes characteristic of CMV IP.

With the exception of rare infectious forms of IP caused by varicella-zoster or herpes simplex virus, *Candida albicans*, Aspergillus, *Pneumocystis carinii*, Legionella, and mycoplasma no specific therapeutic measures exist for this type of lung complication. The clinical outcome is usually lethal, despite symptomatic therapy including mechanical ventilation for patients who show signs of respiratory insufficiency. Due to its potential importance for therapy, identification of the pathogens always should be attempted at the very first signs of IP.

During recent years, the incidence of IP in allogeneic BMT recipients has decreased worldwide and can now be estimated in the range of 10%. This may predominantly be explained by advances in the prevention of CMV disease and in TBI technologies, although the exact contribution of these advances to the reduced incidence of IP remains to be defined. Another important factor may be the restriction of methotrexate to the immediate posttransplant period. This assumption is supported by the well-established pulmonary toxicity of methotrexate together with

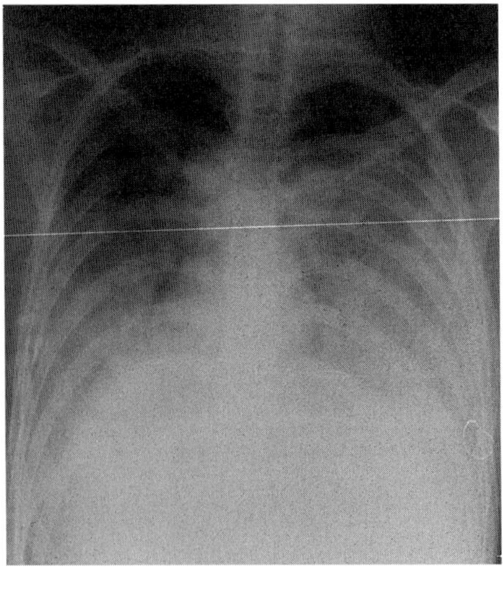

Fig. 12. Chest X-ray of a patient with interstitial pneumonia. (Department of Radiology, University Hospital of Essen.)

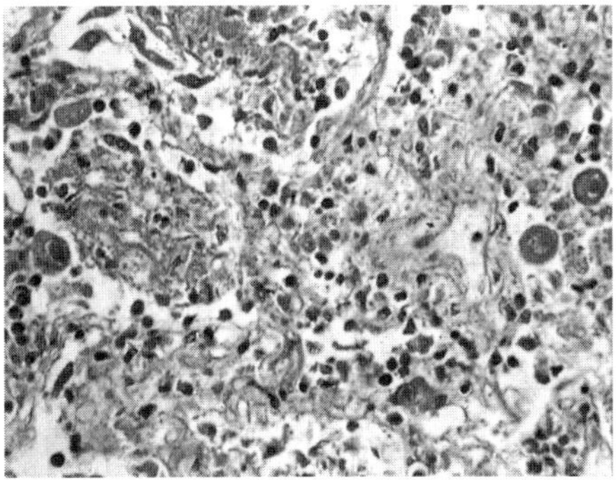

Fig. 13. Histology of CMV interstitial pneumonia (46 days after BMT): Intra-alveolar exudate with fibrin deposits and mononuclear cell infiltrates showing intranuclear CMV inclusions (close to the left and right margin of the picture). HE, × 100. (Department of Pathology, University Hospital of Essen.)

the findings of retrospective analyses that the use of prolonged posttransplant methotrexate was associated with a higher incidence of IP as opposed to ciclosporin A.

8.5. Graft-versus-Host Disease

8.5.1. Acute GvHD

Acute GvHD develops within the first 70 days after allogeneic BMT. The onset of its clinical manifestation is influenced by the degree of disparity between the MHC antigens of the marrow donor and the recipient. After HLA-genotypically identical transplants, the median time interval to the first symptoms is in the range of 20 days posttransplant, which typically coincides with the increase in peripheral blood cell counts. After HLA-partially matched family donor transplants or matched unrelated donor transplants this time interval is about 1 week shorter, and symptoms of acute GvHD may already develop during marrow aplasia in these settings. In contrast, first manifestations of acute GvHD during marrow aplasia or after complete reconstitution of peripheral blood cell parameters are uncommon, if donor and recipient are HLA-genotypically identical siblings.

The incidence of clinically significant (grades II–IV) acute GvHD after HLA-genotypically identical sibling transplantation is in the range of 40–45%, according to the majority of reports from single institutions and transplant registries. After transplantation of marrow from partially HLA-compatible family members, this incidence increases with the number of mismatched HLA-A, -B, -DR antigens of the non-shared haplotype. Besides the crucial importance of disparities of the histocompatibility antigens, which clearly are the most important determining factor for this immunological reaction, retrospective analyses have revealed other factors which influence the development of acute GvHD. Male recipients of grafts from female donors have a significantly increased risk to develop acute GvHD as compared to other gender combinations. Female marrow donors, who have had previous pregnancies or blood transfusions, seem to further increase the risk of acute GvHD in male recipients. This finding supports that alloimmunization against non-MHC-encoded histocompatibility antigens (minor histocompatibility antigens) plays an important role in the pathogenesis of acute GvHD after HLA-genotypically identical transplantation. Further, an increased incidence of acute GvHD with advancing patient or donor age has been repeatedly reported, but this observation is not without contention. As a hypothetical explanation for an increased risk of acute GvHD with advancing patient age, deterioration of the thymic function as a consequence of age involution of the thymus has been suggested. This could be associated with a decreased ability of the thymus to eliminate alloreactive T cells. In a retrospective analysis of the IBMTR, which included 2,036 patients after HLA-identical sibling marrow transplantation, the adverse effect of patient or donor age on the risk of acute GvHD was corroborated in a multivariate analysis after adjustment for the effect of transplants from alloimmunized female donors to male recipients.

Animal experiments and clinical data in patients with SAA after HLA-identical sibling BMT have demonstrated that a germ-free environment in conjunction with bacterial gastrointestinal decontamination is effective in preventing acute GvHD. The mechanisms behind this protective effect are currently not precisely defined. It has been suggested that cross-reactions between cell-wall antigens of intestinal bacteria and histocompatibility antigens may lead to nonspecific stimulation of alloreactive lymphocytes of the marrow graft. Alternatively, soluble products of the intestinal microflora, like bacterial toxins, could lead to an antigen-independent activation of the grafted lymphocytes with a resulting increase in the secretion of lymphokines involved in the propagation of acute GvHD. The value of total gastrointestinal decontamination and a germ-free environment in the prevention of acute GvHD in leukemia patients has so far not been demonstrated in prospective studies.

Current immunogenetic technology is unable to detect differences between minor histocompatibility antigens, which are assumed to be responsible for the development of acute GvHD after HLA-genotypically identical sibling BMT. Therefore, an immunopharmacologic prophylaxis to reduce the risk of acute GvHD is generally mandatory.

Based on the results of animal studies, methotrexate (MTX) was predominately used as an immunosuppressive prophylaxis up to the beginning of the 1980s. The "classical" prophylactic schedule consisted of 15 mg/m^2 MTX IV on day 1 and 10 mg/m^2 MTX IV on days 3, 6, 11 and thereafter every week up to day 102 after transplantation. Even if the value of MTX has never been documented by prospective clinical trials, its efficacy can be regarded as proven in light of the high incidence, early appearance and severity of acute GvHD in patients who did not receive any immunoprophylaxis. Important drawbacks to this type of prophylaxis are the hematopoeitic toxicity of MTX, which contributes to a delay of hematopoietic reconstitution, as well as its toxic effects on mucous membranes, lungs, and the liver.

In contrast to the nonspecific cytotoxic effects of MTX, ciclosporin A specifically inhibits T-cell proliferation, interleukin-2 production and release. It also causes a reduction in the expression of interleukin-2 receptors on T cells and inhibits differentiation of cytotoxic T cells. In a series of studies, in which the immunoprophylactic efficacies of MTX and ciclosporin A were compared, the incidence of acute GvHD and the outcome of transplantation were comparable with both agents. Prophylactic ciclosporin A administration is usually initiated on the day before transplantation, as intravenous bolus injections or as continuous infusions. The parenteral maintenance dose of ciclosporin A is in the range of 3 mg/kg body weight. When the gastrointestinal problems (vomiting, diarrhea, malabsorption) of the early posttransplant phase have subsided, this agent is usually switched to oral application. Due to the intra- and interindividual variations of ciclosporin A absorption, dose adjustments may be necessary according to results of monitoring of ciclosporin A blood levels. Particularly important is the nephrotoxicity of ciclosporin A, which causes a decrease in renal blood flow and glomerular filtration rates leading to elevated creatinine and blood urea-nitrogen concentrations. Close follow-up of renal function parameters and ciclosporin A blood levels is necessary during outpatient care to allow rapid dose adjustments whenever indicated. Ciclosporin A nephrotoxicity is especially critical in combination with other nephrotoxic agents frequently used after BMT, like aminoglycosides, amphotericin B, or ganciclovir. Other frequent adverse effects of ciclosporin A include systemic hypertension, liver dysfunction with cholestasis, fluid retention, central nervous system disturbances, and tremors of varying intensity. Long-term therapy often leads to pronounced hirsutism, which the female patients affected can find to be very annoying. Prophylactic applications of ciclosporin A usually last 6–12 months after transplantation, even though its prophylactic efficacy with regard to chronic GvHD has not yet been definitively proven.

In the mid 1980s, a regimen for prevention of acute GvHD has been developed in Seattle in which MTX on days 1, 3 , 6 and 11 after transplantation (referred to as short-course MTX) was combined with ciclosporin A. In two comparative prospective trials including patients with acute myeloid leukemia (AML) in first remission or in the chronic phase of chronic myeloid leukemia (CML), this combination led to a significant decrease in the incidence and severity of acute GvHD, to a reduction in lethal infectious complications in patients with acute GvHD, and to a significant improvement in the survival probabilities, compared to leukemia patients who received ciclosporin A alone. This combination was further demonstrated to reduce the incidence and severity of acute GvHD and improve survival in patients with SAA as compared to MTX prophylaxis. The superior prophylactic efficacy of short-course MTX and ciclosporin A has further been demonstrated in the HLA-mismatched setting. This combined immunopharmacologic prophylaxis is now broadly accepted as the standard regimen for the prevention of acute GvHD. Combinations of either MTX or ciclosporin A with other immunosuppressive agents, such as prednisone, antithymocyte globulin or T-cell-specific monoclonal antibodies, did not show any convincing reduction in the incidence of acute GvHD when compared to MTX or ciclosporin A alone.

Since mature alloreactive T lymphocytes of the graft apparently play an important role in the development of acute GvHD, several treatment centers have attempted to prevent acute GvHD by decreasing the amount of T cells in the graft. Techniques of ex vivo T-cell depletion are mostly based on monoclonal antibodies directed against antigens expressed on the cell surface of T lymphocytes, which have been coupled to magnetic particles, heterologous erythrocytes, immune absorption columns or toxins, and thus allow a selective elimination of these cells. Other methods are based on complement-dependent cytolytic reactions using polyspecific or monoclonal antibodies in conjunction with human or heterologous complement, or on the physical properties of lymphocytes. Depending on the method chosen, T cells in the graft can be reduced to 0.1–1% of the original amount. In spite of the impressive reduction in the total incidence of acute GvHD to 5–20% using these techniques, transplantation with T-cell-depleted marrow has not improved the overall probability of survival, since reduction of the risk of GvHD was accompanied by an increased graft rejection rate. After HLA-genotypically identical transplantation with nonmanipulated marrow, the graft rejection rate is well under 1%. In contrast, rejection rates of 15–35% have been described by various groups after T-cell-depleted BMT. The risk of rejection further increases, when T-cell depletion is performed in settings of HLA-partially matched transplants. It has further become clear that the risk of relapse in patients with leukemic diseases is increased after T-cell-depleted transplantation. In particular, among patients with CML, relapse rates of up to 75% after transplantation with T-cell-depleted marrow have been reported. In addition, the number of patients with persistent recipient-type hematopoiesis after T-cell-depleted transplants has been shown to be increased. These disadvantages resulted in an inferior outcome of patients after T-cell-depleted as opposed to nonmanipulated BMT. As long as the problems of graft rejection and the increased risk of relapse after T-cell depletion remain unsolved, this highly effective form of acute GvHD prevention has to be regarded as experimental.

Target organs of acute GvHD are the skin, the liver, and the gastrointestinal tract. Characteristically, initial clinical symptoms are skin changes, not uncommonly in the form of itching erythematous-macular rashes on the palms of the hands and soles of the feet (fig. 14), as well as small, spotted, confluent efflorescences on the body trunk, the extremities and the face. In more advanced forms, an extremely painful generalized erythroderma can appear, which may develop into bullous eruptions and exfoliation of the epidermis. This phase has similarities with burn lesions and is accompanied by pronounced exudation and tendency to bacterial superinfection. In some patients the clinical symptoms of acute GvHD are limited to the skin.

Liver involvement is clinically reflected in a cholestatic jaundice, in which the cholestatic enzymes are often substantially raised, while transaminases only show uncharacteristic changes. Bilirubin serum concentrations serve as a measure of liver involvement with acute GvHD. Acute fulminant liver failure accompanied by ascites, encephalopathy and hemorrhagic diathesis resulting from clotting disorders is rare. Recognition of hyperbilirubinemia and of elevated liver enzymes as hepatic involvement with acute GvHD is sometimes difficult, since an unequivocal differentiation between liver impairment resulting from therapy-associated hepatotoxicity, liver changes due to infections, or hepatic VOD is not always possible.

Involvement of the gastrointestinal tract primarily manifests as increased motility, with watery diarrhea. The enteral fluid loss is used as a measure of gastrointestinal involvement with acute GvHD. Advanced disease can be accompanied by severe cramping abdominal pains, sometimes bloody diarrhea and enteral fluid losses of up to 20 l per day, release of mucous membranes, massive entaral protein loss due to protein exudation in the intestinal lumen, and finally intestinal atony with paralytic ileus. As in all clinical symptoms of acute GvHD, gastrointestinal symptoms are nonspecific and must be distinguished from other infectious and toxic intestinal impairments. Isolated liver or enteral involvement without accompanying skin manifestations is unusual and requires, when possible, bioptic prove for diagnostic certainty.

Further concomitant signs of acute GvHD can include fever, tachycardia, decrease in performance status, and weight loss. Clinical staging of organ involvement and the grading of acute GvHD are summarized in table 14. The prognostic signifi-

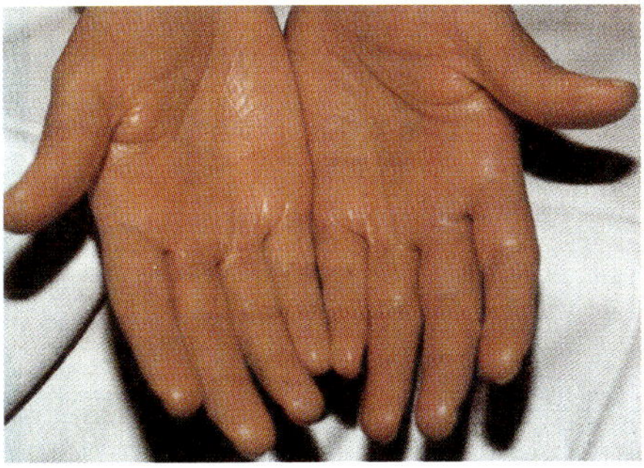

Fig. 14. Characteristic skin reactions of the palms caused by acute GvHD.

Table 14. Clinical stages according to organ system and overall clinical grading of severity of acute GvHD[1]

Stage	Skin	Liver	Intestinal tract
0	no rash	bilirubin, <2 mg/100 ml	<500 ml diarrhea/day
+	maculopapular rash <25 % of body surface	bilirubin, 2–3 mg/100 ml	>500 ml diarrhea/day
++	maculopapular rash 25–50 % of body surface	bilirubin, 3–6 mg/100 ml	>1,000 ml diarrhea/day
+++	generalized erythroderma	bilirubin, 6–15 mg/100 ml	>1,500 ml diarrhea/day
++++	generalized erythroderma with bullous formation and desquamation	bilirubin, >15 mg/100 ml	severe abdominal pain with or without ileus

Grade	Degree of organ involvement
I	+ to ++ skin rash; no gut involvement; no liver involvement; no decrease in clinical performance
II	+ to +++ skin rash; + gut involvement or + liver involvement (or both); mild decrease in clinical performance
III	++ to +++ skin rash; ++ to +++ gut involvement or ++ to ++++ liver involvement (or both); marked decrease in clinical performance
IV	similar to grade III with ++ to ++++ organ involvement and extreme decrease in clinical performance

[1] Thomas et al: New Engl J Med 1975; 292:832–895.

cance of the clinical degree of severity is best reflected in the increased mortality of patients who develop grades II–IV acute GvHD.

Histologic skin changes of acute GvHD are characterized by infiltrations of mononuclear cells, vacuolization of basal cells, and single-cell necrosis of epithelial cells, which are occasionally surrounded by lymphocytes (fig. 15). More pronounced involvement leads to larger necrotic areas and exfoliation of the epidermis.

Liver tissue predominantly changes around the bile ducts and is characterized by degeneration of the small ducts in the form of segmental necrosis, with a characteris-

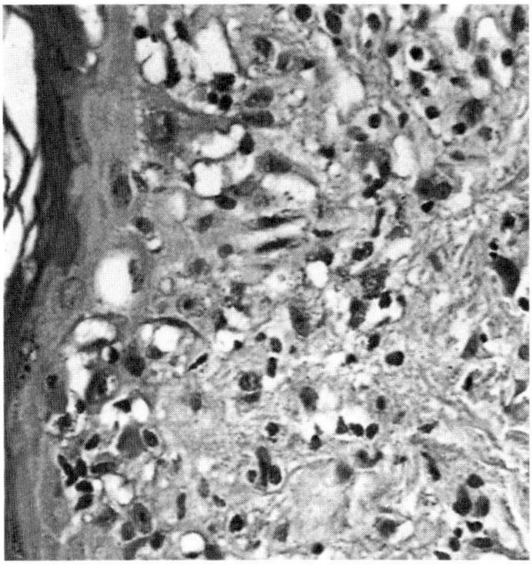

Fig. 15. Histology of acute GvHD of the skin: Lymphocytic infiltrates of the upper dermis and epidermis. Hydropic vacuolar degeneration of basal cells. Single eosinophilic necrotic changes of keratinocytes. HE × 100. (Department of Pathology, University Hospital of Essen.)

tic cytoplasmatic eosinophilia of bile-duct cells. Periportal fields can appear spread out due to lymphocyte infiltration.

In mild acute GvHD, the intestinal mucous membranes show single-cell necrosis around the basal crypts surrounded by lymphocyte infiltration. Inflammatory infiltration can disseminate over the entire mucous membrane and lead to crypt abscesses, inflamed ulcers, and desquamation of the epithelium.

Immunosuppressants are used as therapy for acute GvHD and in the majority of patients, lead to an improvement or complete suppression of acute symptoms. The most extensive experience has been with corticosteroids which, depending on the severity of clinical symptoms and therapeutic response, are given in a dose ranging from 2 mg/kg body weight to a total daily dose of 2 g. Other immunosuppressants used either alone or in combinations for the treatment of acute GvHD are ciclosporin A, antithymocyte globulin, cyclophosphamide and, more recently, T-cell-specific monoclonal antibodies. Other important supportive measures besides immunosuppression, particularly in the initial phase of treatment, are parenteral hyperalimentation in cases of malabsorption, replacement therapy of enteral losses of fluids, proteins and electrolytes, preventive measures against infections, and timely institution of antibiotic therapy whenever infections are suspected or documented. Treatment of GvHD generally takes several months and has to be adjusted to each patient individually according to the therapeutic response and the sequelae of nonspecific immunosuppression. In spite of the often satisfactory response of acute symptoms, the indispensable immunosuppression used to treat GvHD is coupled with problems which have a decisive impact on the prognosis of this complication. The most prominent of these is the immunodeficiency inherent in acute GvHD, further aggravated by the immunosuppressive therapy. This results in pronounced susceptibility to various infectious complications. Despite all preventive measures, viral infections as well as late manifestations of bacterial and mycotic infections are the most common cause of death in patients with acute or secondary chronic GvHD. Impairment of specific cellular immunity facilitate, above all, the reactivation of latent CMV infections or other herpesvirus infections. CMV IP represents therefore a major cause of death in patients with acute GvHD. 50% of patients who develop acute GvHD of grades II-IV die of infections within the first 2 years after transplantation.

8.5.2. Chronic GvHD

Chronic GvHD can occur anytime within the 1st year after transplantation. In general, symptoms of chronic GvHD do not develop before day 100, in exceptional cases around day 70. The total incidence of chronic GvHD is about 30–50% in patients surviving longer than 6 months after HLA-identical sibling BMT. In the majority of patients affected, the symptoms of chronic GvHD appear either after an asymptomatic interval or immediately following acute GvHD (referred to as secondary chronic GvHD). In 20–30% of patients, however, chronic GvHD is the first clinical manifestation of histoincompatibility. Acute GvHD is the major determining factor for the development of chronic GvHD. Depending on the degree of organ involvement, two clinical courses of chronic GvHD can be distinguished: limited chronic GvHD consists of localized skin manifestations and/or mild liver function impairment; extensive chronic GvHD involves generalized skin manifestations, or localized skin manifestations in conjunction with more severe liver involvement, involvement of salivary glands, or other organ systems (table 15).

The clinical appearance of chronic GvHD shows some similarities with a number of collagen-vascular diseases such as Sjögren's syndrome, localized or systemic sclerodermia, lichen planus, systemic lupus erythematodes or primary biliary cirrhosis. Contrary to sclerodermia, chronic GvHD is not accompanied by fibrosis in the smooth muscles of the esophagus or involvement of the myenteric plexus. Kidney involvement, common in lupus erythematodes or sclerodermia, is not seen in chronic GvHD, and development of liver cirrhosis and portal hypertension as a consequence of hepatic involvement is uncommon with chronic GvHD.

Most patients with chronic GvHD show skin manifestations of generalized or localized bright red edematous patches, as well as desquamatous and scaly skin lesions (fig. 16). Secondary changes include atrophy of the epidermis, thickening and sclerosis of the subcutis, and trophic impairment of hair and nails. These changes can be so pronounced in untreated patients that joint contractures result.

Table 15. Clinical grading of chronic GvHD[1]

Limited chronic GvHD
Either or both:
1. Localized skin involvement
2. Hepatic dysfunction due to chronic GvHD
Extensive chronic GvHD
Either:
1. Generalized skin involvement;
or
2. Localized skin involvement and/or hepatic dysfunction due to chronic GvHD, plus:
3. a. Liver histology showing chronic aggressive hepatitis, bridging necrosis, or cirrhosis;
or
b. Involvement of eye (Schirmer's test with <5 mm wetting);
or
c. Involvement of minor salivary glands or oral mucosa demonstrated on labial biopsy;
or
d. Involvement of any other organ

[1] Shulman et al: Am J Med (1980); 69: 204

Involvement of the oral mucous membranes, which is observed in over 80% of patients with disseminated chronic GvHD, manifests primarily as a lichenoid reaction at the cheeks and tongue, characterized by striped, reticular or large plaque-like changes. Usually atrophy of the mucous membranes is accompanied by reduced keratinization and xerostomy, which promote the development of severe parodontosis and caries. Due to the involvement of the salivary and lacrimal glands, the majority of patients with disseminated chronic GvHD develop sicca syndrome. This makes artificial tear fluid replacement necessary and can further lead to recurrent keratoconjunctivitis.

Liver involvement is reflected in increased plasma bilirubin and enzyme levels, in which a pattern either of liver parenchymal damage or of cholestasis can predominate. Involvement of the esophagus is typical and can be accompanied by motility impairment and stenosis, leading to dysphagic symptoms and retrosternal pain. Additional symptoms of chronic GvHD, especially in untreated patients, include weight loss, malabsorption, recurrent infections, and joint contractures.

Early histopathological changes in the skin during disseminated chronic GvHD show up as hypertrophy and hyperkeratosis of the epidermis, with accompanying lichenoid reaction and vacuolic degeneration of the basal skin layers, edema in the area of the papillar stratum and lympho-plasmacellular infiltrations of the hair follicles and subcutis. Immunohistology shows deposits of immunoglobulins and com-

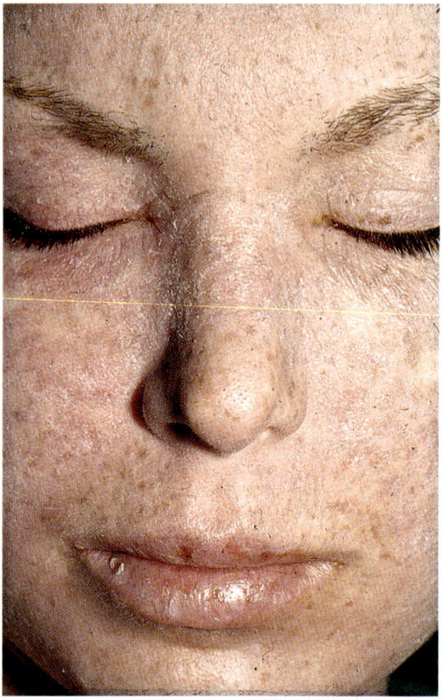

Fig. 16. Characteristic skin lesions of chronic GvHD.

plement in the transitional zone between dermis and epidermis. In advanced chronic GvHD, fibrotic changes and atrophy of the epidermis predominate. In localized chronic GvHD, these changes seem to develop first. Histological changes in the liver found in chronic GvHD are similar to those described for acute GvHD and depend in their intensity on the duration and degree of active liver involvement. The histological picture can resemble chronic aggressive hepatitis and is generally characterized by the presence of cholestatic changes and vanishing of the small bile ducts. The salient histological characteristics of other epithelial tissue involvement, as well as salivary or lacrimal glands involvement, are mononuclear cell infiltrations, epithelial cell necrosis, and fibrotic alterations.

The prognosis of patients with chronic GvHD is substantially influenced by two factors:

1. the clinical course – patients with limited chronic GvHD have a much better prognosis than those with extensive chronic GvHD;
2. the time of appearance and its relation to a preceding acute GvHD.

Patients who develop secondary chronic GvHD immediately following acute GvHD have the worst prognosis, and patients with de novo chronic GvHD have the most favorable one. Thus, the most effective prophylaxis for chronic GvHD is to prevent acute GvHD. At present, the different strategies of immunopharmacologic prophylaxis have not reliably demonstrated effectiveness in preventing the development of chronic GvHD.

Patients with disseminated chronic GvHD receive monotherapy with prednisone in a daily oral dose of 1–2 mg/kg. In cases of insufficient therapeutic response, combination therapy can be attempted using azathioprine, ciclosporin A, procarbazine or cyclophosphamide in addition to prednisone. Although combination therapy using prednisone and azathioprine was more effective in suppressing the symptoms of disease when compared to prednisone alone in a randomized trial, it increased the rate of infectious complications, and the survival of patients was adversely affected. Further, there is growing evidence that the use of azathioprine is burdened by an increased risk of secondary cancers in patients with chronic GvHD. Results from comparative trials suggest that the combination of ciclosporin A and alternate-day prednisone can improve the outcome of patients with extensive chronic GvHD. Nevertheless, the choice of immunosuppressive strategy for each patient with disseminated chronic GvHD has largely to rely on the expertise of the transplant physician and has to be modified on an individual basis in many affected patients. As with acute GvHD, supportive therapy such as artificial tear fluid replacement in cases of ocular sicca syndrome, strict compliance to hygienic measures, use of prophylactic antibiotics, early initiation of antibiotic chemotherapy in cases of suspected or proven infections, and physiotherapy to prevent joint contractures may be of crucial importance for survival and quality of life of patients suffering from chronic GvHD.

8.6. Leukemic Relapse after BMT

The reappearance of leukemia after BMT depends, above all, on the stage of disease at the time of transplantation. This reflects the increasing resistance of hematologic neoplasias to the radiochemotherapeutic conditioning treatment with advancing disease. The increased relapse rates after syngeneic transplantation as well as the reduced incidence of relapses among patients who develop acute or chronic GvHD suggest an immunologic antileukemic component in allogeneic transplantation–also referred to as graft-versus-leukemia effect–which is independent of the tumoricidal effect of the conditioning treatment.

Typically, leukemic relapse occurs within the first 2–3 years after transplantation. However, isolated cases of relapse have been described more than 6 years after allogeneic transplants. In the majority of patients who survive the first 3 years after transplantation without leukemic recurrence, it can be assumed that a definite cure of the underlying disease has been achieved.

Up to now, it remains uncertain whether prognostic factors which determine the probability of relapse after conventional chemotherapy in patients with acute leukemia are also applicable to the relapse risk after allogeneic transplantation. If the prognostic significance of these factors was reduced or abolished in recipients of allogeneic BMTs, especially patients with a higher relapse risk after conventional therapy might benefit from the superior antileukemic effect of allogeneic BMT. A number of prospective comparative studies addressing this unresolved issue are currently performed.

With the aim of increasing the antileukemic efficacy of the standard radiochemotherapeutic conditioning protocol, numerous clinical trials have been performed using combinations of various cytotoxic agents with cyclophosphamide and TBI. Further, different TBI schedules with varying fractionations, dose rates, and total doses have been investigated. In spite of promising data from generally small, uncontrolled trials, there is at present no evidence that current modifications of the radiochemotherapeutic conditioning therapy substantially reduce leukemic relapse rates after allogeneic transplantation without an acceptable increase in regimen-related toxicities. Most importantly, none of these numerous modifications of the conditioning regimen has yet provided evidence of a reduction in the risk of relapse combined with an improvement of survival probability, when compared to the standard combination of cyclophosphamide and TBI.

The relapse probabilities after allogeneic BMT as a function of the disease stage at transplantation show remarkable consistency in all large-scale analyses. In AML, the relapse probability for patients treated in first CR is given in the range of 20–25%. Relapse probabilities increase in untreated first relapse or in second CR to 40%, and in more advanced disease stages to 60%. The corresponding figures for acute lymphoblastic leukemia (ALL) are in first CR 25–35% for patients fulfilling high-risk criteria at diagnosis, in second CR about 45% for standard-risk patients compared to about 55% in high-risk patients, and in more advanced disease stages up to 75% (high-risk criteria according to an IBMTR analysis: patients older than 16 years, white blood cell counts in excess of 50×10^9/l, FAB-L3 subtype, B phenotype, central nervous system involvement, and chromosomal aberrations). A retrospective analysis by the IBMTR suggests that, at least in patients with ALL in second CR, these prognostic criteria are associated with a higher relapse risk both after conventional chemotherapy and after allogeneic BMT.

In patients with acute leukemia, the definitive diagnosis of relapse is usually based on morphological criteria. In patients with CML, a distinction is made between the reappearance or persistence of Philadelphia chromosome-positive

(Ph+) cells as demonstrated by cytogenetic or molecular genetic techniques and a hematologic relapse diagnosed on the basis of the typical morphological pattern of CML in peripheral blood and bone marrow. The probability of hematologic relapse in patients in the first chronic phase is about 20%, and this increases in the accelerated phase or in the phase of acute transformation to 50–80%. For the small number of patients in acute transformation who achieve a second chronic phase after conventional chemotherapy, the probability of relapse is clearly reduced as compared to patients who received transplants in the overt blastic phase of CML. The significance of single Ph+ cells observed in cytogenetic follow-up examinations after transplantation remains unclear at present. It is not uncommon to observe single Ph+ cells in the early phase after transplantation. Also, during the first years after transplantation, Ph+ cells have repeatedly been described without the subsequent development of hematologic relapse of CML. However, it must still be assumed that an initially high or increasing percentage of Ph+ cells after transplantation, even when the bone marrow morphology is normal, indicates an incipient hematologic relapse. Follow-up examinations on a larger number of patients with persisting or reappearing Ph+ cells in conjunction with other markers of hematopoietic chimaeras will be needed to clearly determine the risk of hematologic relapse in patients with reappearance of cytogenetically defined disease posttransplant. During recent years, monitoring of bcr/abl transcripts by the PCR has become an important tool for the detection of minimal residual disease in patients with Ph+ CML in the posttransplant course. There is growing evidence that follow-up studies using this diagnostic tool can be used to define a population of patients with a substantially increased relapse risk. This method may thus provide the basis for studies of early therapeutic interventions in patients with minimal residual disease after allogeneic BMT, like the application of interferon-α or of donor buffy-coat transfusions.

9. Allogeneic Bone Marrow Transplantation Using Volunteer-Unrelated Bone Marrow Donors

An increasing number of transplantations have now been performed using donors other than HLA-identical siblings, including HLA-partially matched family donors and partially or fully matched unrelated donors. Results of transplants using related donors sharing only one HLA haplotype are poor. If two additional antigens are phenotypically identical between the nonidentical HLA haplotypes of related donor-recipient pairs, the outcome of such transplantations is not significantly different from those of HLA-identical sibling transplantations.

About 65–70% of patients in Europe and North America who are potential candidates for a marrow allograft lack an HLA-identical sibling. The use of unrelated donors thus has the potential to extend the availability of BMT to the majority of patients who might benefit from an allogeneic BMT. It has been calculated that a donor pool size of 100,000 to 1,000,000 individuals would yield HLA-A-, -B-, -DR-phenotypically identical donors for about 50–75% of Caucasian patients with common HLA haplotypes.

In recent years, a rapidly increasing number of transplantations with unrelated donors have been performed, predominantly in patients with CML, but also in patients with AAL, SAA, and severe combined immunodeficiency syndromes.

Current experience indicates that the incidences of acute and chronic GvHD are clearly increased after HLA-matched unrelated donor transplantations compared to HLA-matched sibling BMT. While the risk of graft failure does not seem to be substantially higher, other transplantation-associated complications like pulmonary toxicity as well as early and late infectious complications appear to be more common among recipients of marrow from unrelated donors. Results from an international comparative trial (IMUST) indicate that with current techniques of marrow grafting the results of HLA-matched unrelated marrow donor transplantations are significantly inferior to those of HLA-matched sibling transplantations.

With growing donor pool sizes, advances in histocompatibility testing and donor selection, and in the techniques of BMT it can be expected that the wide investments in unrelated donor programs worldwide will provide sufficiently matched donors to the majority of patients together with a reasonably save therapeutic procedure.

10. Psychosocial Problems Associated with Allogeneic Bone Marrow Transplantation

Jürgen Neuser

BMT is a form of therapy that makes great demands on the patient. The decision to undergo BMT is made with the knowledge that it offers the best existing possibility of a cure, but at the same time carries with it a high risk of mortality. The period of transplantation is associated with greatly restricted freedom of movement. The treatment itself is gruelling and can have grave side effects, yet relies on a substantial amount of patient compliance. Life after transplantation is, at first, full of limitations, including long-term dependency on medical care. Persisting late sequelae are not fully known, and in individual cases the success of treatment cannot be reliably determined beforehand. This list should be enough to illustrate the psychological stress in which the patient finds himself. Not only for the patient himself, but also for his or her significant others, for the bone marrow donor, and for the team of doctors and nurses, BMT poses a host of psychological difficulties. Research into psychological problems related to BMT is still relatively unsystematic and leaves many questions open. The current findings are given here, and are supplemented with personal experience in the psychological supervision of BMT patients, where empirical data are lacking.

10.1. Psychosocial Problems of BMT Patients

In small children, the fundamental concern is the possibility that developmental retardation could be induced. In most cases this problem can be avoided when an ersatz mother is available during the hospital stay. In addition to transient instances of psychopathologic symptoms (jactation, regurgitation, etc.), impairment of speech development in small children has to be expected if the necessary encouragement to speak is not provided.

School-age children are often able to comprehend and understand the necessity for treatment. This, however, leads to the emergence of obvious emotional problems. At this age, fear and anxiety are common problems. A good relationship between the child and the doctor or other health care professionals and, in cases of pronounced fear, behavior-oriented psychotherapy, can contribute to a reduction of fear. Depression, also in association with regressive and aggressive behavior, is observed in about 10% of children and is a common cause of cooperation problems.

Other problems are not seen more frequently than in hospitalized children in general. Even at the time of admission to hospital for BMT, these children exhibit poorer school performance than their healthy contemporaries, in spite of an average IQ. This tendency can be expected to become worse during the BMT.

In puberty, psychologically based inhibitions, which develop following changes in outward appearance, become important. During clinical treatment, adolescent patients react more strongly to (perceived) intrusions in their sphere of intimacy and attempt to mark off their personal space in various ways. Here it is necessary to be very tactful in dealing with the patient's sphere of intimacy. After release from hospital quite a few young (teenage) patients have psychological problems such as fear of being disfigured or marred, social isolation, and depression. On the other hand, many adolescent BMT patients, when compared to those treated with chemotherapy, have a more positive attitude toward life in general, better social skills, and greater faith in the eventual realization of their personal plans.

Adult BMT patients suffer psychosocial problems, in addition to the period involved with the transplantation itself (decision to undergo the transplantation, waiting for the necessary arrangements to be made, the transplantation itself, and the posttransplant period). Only retrospective data are available on the decision and waiting periods. Hardly any patient whose doctor recommends a BMT as possible treatment rejects it. After receiving detailed information, patients, nearly without exception, decide within a few days in favor of transplantation. Hereby, it should be added, there is reason to assume that doctors contribute to a preselection bias, based on the psychosocial characteristics of the patient. Among our patients with leukemia, those who showed a strong sense of perseverance and discipline were overrepresented. Since it can be assumed that leukemia patients do not differ from the total population in the frequency of these characteristics, it has to be surmised that the referring doctors implicitly assume that perseverance and discipline are necessary for successful BMT. In our study, however, these characteristics did not correlate with the success of treatment.

The process of deciding to undergo transplantation often implies the assignment of responsibility for the decision within the family, which occasionally can give rise to conflict.

The waiting period after the decision is, for many patients, a time of inner tension, in the nature of a double ambivalence conflict: On the one side, there is the hope that the illness can be controlled without BMT, and on the other the fear of relapse or crisis; then there is the hope that BMT will prevent progression of the primary disease, and the fear that the disease cannot be controlled even with BMT. Admission to hospital is then experienced as relief.

For clinicians the psychosocial problems of the transplantation period are of particular interest. The available reports are predominantly case histories of the psychological supervision of BMT patients. In Essen, we had the opportunity to perform the first prospective longitudinal study on leukemia patients. We attempted to identify the components of psychological stress and how they developed over time. These components were extracted, using a statistical method (principle component analysis), from patient self-reports about their immediate feelings and from reports of medical attendants about medically relevant psychological problems like cooperation, nausea and vomiting, and sleep problems. The result was four stress components, which can be characterized as "Emotional Distress", "Physical Distress", "Tension" and "Hostility/Aversion". The varying intensities of these stress components during the course of the transplantation period show that different qualities of distress dominate at different points of time. Overall psychological distress is greatest at the time of aplasia, but greater tension and anger reactions can be expected when the patient is in comparatively good physical shape.

Severe depression and psychotic episodes occur in about 8% of BMT patients and should be treated with medication. They coincide, in nearly all cases, with severe transplantation related complications.

What is experienced during the transplantation period influences psychosocial convalescence, so that early attention to psychological problems is indicated. The psychosocial situation 2 years after transplantation is satisfactory for the majority of patients. Fear and cognitive impairment, however, are more pronounced than in comparable groups of bone marrow donors and do not show a tendency to diminish with time after release from hospital.

10.2. Psychosocial Problems of Bone Marrow Donors

Up to now, only one article about the psychosocial problems of adult bone marrow donors has been published. With the exception of only a few cases, it can be said that donating has a positive influence on the donors' feelings of self-esteem and that for most people donation of bone marrow is not accompanied by psychosocial problems. Just as donation can sometimes result in resolution of conflicts – for example, the donor who felt responsible for the accidental death of a sibling in her childhood, and who experienced donating bone marrow as kind of atonement –, donation can under certain circumstances also revive psychological conflicts. When the possibility exists to choose between more than one donor, these aspects should be taken into consideration.

When the donors are children, psychological problems are more prevalent. The removal of bone marrow can awaken archaic fears, fear of death, fear of killing, punishment fantasies, and poison fantasies. These fears can develop subtly, and often remain unnoticed at first. For this reason children need the attention of mental health professionals when they donate bone marrow.

10.3. Psychosocial Problems of Significant Others

The BMT patient's significant others are involved in the tension surrounding treatment. Since many patients live far away from the treatment center, the first consequence of BMT is the disruption of the family context. Taking over the partner's functions and roles, caring for dependent family members, as well as the time taken up with hospital visits, often in addition to regular employment, represent additional strain which is unrelated to the course of treatment. The financial burden of BMT should also not be underestimated.

The psychosocial problems of significant others of adult BMT patients have not yet been the subject of scientific investigation. Patients regard family members as the principle source of social support. Friends and others play a lesser role during the transplantation period. The stress a patient experiences is particularly high when he or she comes from an intact family context. According to preliminary results of a study we have begun, the psychological burden of significant others is comparable in intensity to that of the patient. However, it seems that there is a difference in the length and type of events that patients and significant others perceive as burdensome. Significant others are particularly put off by a patient's depressive mood, by communication problems resulting from stomatitis, and men are disturbed by changes in their wives' outward appearance. Also the psychological burden to significant others of multiple tasks, sleeplessness (sitting with the patient through the night), or insomnia should not be underestimated.

For parents and siblings of children who are to receive BMTs, the search for a donor is the most stressful occurrence of the waiting period. At the time of admission for BMT, 70% of mothers and fathers show signs of depression. During treatment, symptoms of exhaustion and insomnia increase. Parents' perception of their marital relationship was not found to be different from that of parents of healthy children. Brothers and sisters often develop behavior problems.

After the patient has been discharged from hospital, many families have to deal with problems of reintegration into the family circle. In some cases, tension results from drastic demands on the partner to change certain habits and thus make a new beginning possible. Reintegration efforts, however, have to be undertaken by all families.

10.4. Psychosocial Problems of the Treatment Team

BMT is a form of intensive care medicine and therefore similar phenomena are found in BMT wards as in other areas of intensive-medicine. Coping with emotional strain and role conflicts are frequently mentioned stress factors of the attending health care professionals, and can lead to excessive personal involvement, close personal contact outside working hours, and a high rate of personnel turnover. The psychosocial problems of doctors are in principle similar but, in addition, decisions which carry weighty consequences have to be dealt with. Since many patients are in good physical condition when they come to the transplantation center, doctors in BMT wards are perhaps under greater psychological pressure "to bring the patient through". The hopes raised by BMT cannot remain without consequences in this respect, either.

10.5. When Patients Die

During the transplantation period a close relationship develops between the patient and the treatment team. For this reason, the treatment team also goes through a period of mourning when a patient dies. Each patient demands commitment and emotional investment, which are rewarded by the patient's recovery. The death of the patient makes these efforts pointless and places the entire endeavor in question.

This aspect is also important for the significant others, who have to restructure their emotional ties to the deceased. The let-down, which corresponds in intensity to the hope which preceded it, can sometimes lead to complaints and accusations against the treatment team. Not uncommonly, comments are made which do not seem to be in keeping with grief over the death, such as the mention of a future with a new partner. Comments like these meet with rejection and repulsion, but should be understood as momentary expressions of despair, rage at being abandoned, and deep disappointment. They are components of every mourning reaction.

When children die, the families often need more time to recover from this loss than from the loss of an adult. Even after 2 years, 50% of parents show mourning reactions which have to be regarded as pathologic. About 20% of brothers and sisters develop manifest problems in school, in psychological areas, and in social interaction. There is a connection between the total length of treatment and the persistence of symptoms in parents and siblings of the deceased child.

The patients themselves generally have a very realistic estimation of whether or not they will survive complications. Usually, a process of withdrawal begins which makes it possible to rationally discuss wishes and impending events. The people in the immediate social vicinity, who are doing everything to prevent death, then face the dilemma of wanting to continue their efforts and also of wanting to understand the patient and his emotional situation.

Just as restoration of health and its fulfilment of the hopes of the patient, the significant others and the treatment team are a part of the reality of BMT, so also is dying a part of this reality. BMT, however, is always accompanied by a greater or lesser degree of psychological burden, and patients, as well as others involved, need psychological support.

11. Follow-Up Care after Allogeneic Bone Marrow Transplantation

The final outcome of otherwise successful marrow transplantation is largely determined by complications within the first 6–12 months after discharge from hospital. Early detection and treatment of these complications require comprehensive patient information and a close cooperation between all institutions involved in the follow-up care of marrow transplant patients. During the 1st year after transplantation, viral (primarily through CMV and varicella-zoster virus), bacterial, mycotic and other opportunistic infections as well as chronic GvHD are of crucial prognostic significance. Adequate care of patients with chronic GvHD and its associated secondary complications depends, to a large extent, on sufficient therapeutic experience as well as on adequate understanding of the complex immunobiologic problems. For these reasons, the coordination and implementation of follow-up care should be performed at an appropriate transplantation center. In addition, it is important to monitor the potential adverse effects of immunoprophylactic or therapeutic ciclosporin A treatment, which some centers use over time periods of 9–12 months after transplantation. Late manifestations of IP predominantly occur in total-body-irradiated patients suffering from chronic GvHD, who require immunosuppressive therapy for prolonged time periods.

According to our experience, the first 3 months after discharge from the hospital are particularly critical; therefore we recommend 1- or 2-weekly visits in the outpatient department of the responsible transplantation center during this time period. The aims of these outpatient follow-up visits are prevention, early detection and treatment of therapy-associated adverse effects and infectious complications, and to monitor hematopoietic and immunologic reconstitution. The intensity of follow-up care will largely be determined by the presence or development of chronic GvHD. Patients not suffering from this immunologic complication generally do not pose any particular clinical problem, even though late infections can sporadically occur in this patient group.

After termination of immunoprophylaxis, we regard outpatient visits in 1- to 3-month intervals as sufficient for asymptomatic patients during the 1st posttransplantation year. Patients requiring treatment for chronic GvHD, on the other hand, should come for outpatient visits more frequently. The exact intervals will depend on the response to, and tolerance of, the immunosuppressive therapy. As symptoms subside, the interval between follow-up examinations can increase. As a rule, all patients should receive yearly follow-up examinations for the rest of their lives at the respective transplantation center to permit long-term observations of any possible rare late adverse effects of marrow transplantation.

11.1. Control Examinations at Outpatient Follow-Up Visits

Hematology and Immunology

Hemogram, differential white blood count, reticulocyte count, bone marrow cytology and histology, chromosome and molecular studies for the detection of disease- or individual-specific markers, blood group serology, enzyme polymorphisms, immunophenotyping of leukocytes, immune reactivity (lymphocyte transformation testing using antigen and mitogen stimulation), quantitative immunoglobulin determination, and immune electrophoresis.

Clinical Chemistry

Liver and kidney function parameters, serum electrolytes (including magnesium serum concentration during ciclosporin treatment), haptoglobin, serum protein electrophoresis, ciclosporin A blood level, vitamin B12 and folic acid determinations, FSH, LH, TSH, peripheral estrogen or testosterone concentrations and, in children, growth hormone determination.

Infectology

Bacterial, fungal and viral surveillance cultures. Screening of antibodies against viral, fungal or other opportunistic germs.

Other Examinations

Chest X-ray, pulmonary function analysis, ECG tracings, cardiac and abdominal ultrasound scan.

During the first 3 months following transplantation and as long as an immunosuppressive therapy is necessary, we recommend the following infection-preventive measures to our patients:

1. Antimycotic decontamination of the gastrointestinal tract with a nonabsorbable oral antimycotic agent (amphotericin B, nystatin).
2. Prophylaxis of *Pneumocystis carinii* pneumonia and antibacterial decontamination orally by cotrimoxazole twice weekly.
3. Regular disinfection of the oral mucous membranes and the palms.
4. Regular control of body temperature.

Prophylaxis against exogenous infections:

1. Avoid contact with infected individuals, large gatherings of people (public transportation, department stores, bars, public swimming pools, etc.) and direct body contacts (shaking hands, hugging etc.).
2. Use sanitary facilities which are exclusively provided for the patient and are disinfected daily.
3. No pets (especially no cats or birds).
4. Regular disinfection of the living area, removal of house plants out of the immediate vicinity.
5. Dietetic hygiene (consuming well-balanced meals, freshly prepared food, no unpeeled fruit, no salad, no raw vegetables).

Besides these recommendations, all patients are advised to contact their treatment center immediately if they feel unwell or develop symptoms of infection, in order to arrange appropriate diagnostic or therapeutic intervention. During the first 2 years after transplantation, exposure of the skin to ultraviolet rays has to be avoided at all costs since this can activate alloreactive cells and thus lead to the development of GvHD. Exposed skin areas, therefore, have to be protected from sunlight by using creams with high screening factors. Generally, it is recommended that all patients use a fatty skin cream. It is also important to clean teeth thoroughly and the interdental spaces regularly.

Female patients who received TBI will need hormone replacement therapy as prophylaxis for endocrine ovarian insufficiency for the rest of their lives.

If blood cell substitution is necessary, all blood products should be irradiated with at least 15 Gy to prevent transfusion-induced acute GvHD. In seronegative patients who received marrow grafts from a CMV antibody-negative donor, exclusively blood products from seronegative donors should be given to prevent CMV transmission. If this cannot be performed, high-efficiency depletion of leukocytes from the blood products by leukocyte removal in-line filtration is mandatory.

Patients requiring treatment for chronic GvHD should follow the above mentioned rules until all symptoms of disease are under control and the immunosuppressive therapy can be terminated. Additional prophylactic therapeutic measures recommendable for patients with chronic GvHD include:

1. Antibiotic long-term prophylaxis with oral penicillins.
2. Artificial tear fluid replacement in cases of ocular sicca syndrome.
3. Immunoglobulin substitution in case of secondary immunoglobulin deficiency.
4. Physiotherapy to prevent joint contractures and inactivation atrophies.

The value of passive immunization using CMV hyperimmunoglobulins is not yet established, and thus cannot be generally recommended. On the other hand, primary varicella-zoster (VZV) virus infection appears to be effectively suppressed by hyperimmunoglobulin when immunization is performed within 48 h after exposure. Herpes simplex virus (HSV) disease and VZV disease can be effectively treated with immediate systemic acyclovir therapy. Life-threatening disseminated disease or severe organ manifestations have become rare when this therapy is used. Immunization using attenuated living vaccines has long been regarded as obsolete due to the risks of transmitting disease. Due to reduced immune reactivity, even an inactivated vaccine within the 1st year after transplantation, or in patients receiving immunosuppressive therapy, is not very likely to succeed. In particular, patients with chronic GvHD, who could benefit the most from vaccination, are the least suitable to receive an active immunization, due to their impaired specific cellular immunity. Recent vaccination studies in pediatric BMT patients support that active vaccination may be feasible, although this issue has further to be evaluated in more comprehensive studies including adult patients.

The majority of patients, after the end of the 1st year after transplantation, are able to lead a normal life, so that reintegration into education or profession should be attempted. In individual cases, depending on the type of profession and the amount of physical exertion involved, some limitations or disabilities can result. Even patients requiring treatment for chronic GvHD need not be barred from working if the appropriate hygienic standards are available at the workplace. In patients with extensive chronic GvHD, however, partial or even total employment disability can be assumed. Since allogeneic BMT offers the chance of a definite cure without further treatment, reintegration into working life is, according to our experience, an important component in overcoming the patient's sense of being ill.

12. Autologous Bone Marrow or Blood Progenitor Cell Transplantation

The first report of the retransfusion of a patient's own bone marrow (autologous BMT) goes back to the year 1959. At that time, the application of autologous transplantation in patients with terminal stages of acute lymphoblastic leukemia (ALL), who had been treated with TBI, did not arouse much interest. Developments in the area of allogeneic and syngeneic transplantation since the mid 1970s have stimulated a large number of working groups to reconsider and further develop the concept of autologous transplantation in malignant hematologic systemic diseases and in solid tumors. The number of patients treated with high-dose radiochemotherapy and autologous transplantation is currently dramatically increasing worldwide.

Autologous transplantation is based on the phenomenon that a steep dose-response relationship exists in many radiochemotherapy-sensitive tumors. Dose escalation of most cytotoxic agents, however, is limited by bone marrow toxicity. Potentially irreversible therapy-related damage to the patient's bone marrow can be avoided by removal and cryopreservation of bone marrow stem cells before exposing the patient to high-dose cytotoxic treatment. The retransfusion of these cells following such therapy can lead to a complete reconstitution of bone marrow function. Animal experiments and human data clearly demonstrate that the dose escalation achievable by autologous stem cell support can result in a substantially increased tumor cell kill compared to conventional chemotherapy. This, in turn, can lead to responses in tumors resistant to conventional doses of these agents. Based on preliminary results of phase I/II studies, it is estimated that the maximum tolerable doses of a wide variety of cytotoxic substances can be increased 3- to 8-fold over conventional levels when the dose-limiting bone marrow toxicity can be circumvented.

As a basic principle, only malignant diseases which meet the following criteria should be chosen for this type of therapy:

1. The tumor response should be directly related to the dose of a cytostatic drug or of irradiation.
2. Tumor infiltration of the bone marrow should not be present, or be in occult form, following successful primary therapy.

Tumor entities which generally fulfil these criteria include acute leukemias in CR, intermediate- or high-grade non-Hodgkin's lymphomas as well as Hodgkin's disease, neuroblastoma, breast cancer, ovarian and testicular cancer, small-cell lung cancer, and some soft-tissue sarcomas. Current experience further suggests that sustained response to high-dose therapy can preferably be expected when treatment is carried out in the early disease stages and when tumor mass is low. High-dose therapy necessitating autologous transplantation should therefore preferentially be considered as consolidation therapy following successful primary therapy or as therapy of a sensitive tumor relapse.

Conditioning treatment in leukemias is aimed at killing clonogenic leukemic cells in the bone marrow. However, due to its lack of selectivity, hematopoietic stem cells are invariably destroyed as well. In primary localized or disseminated tumors which are not accompanied by bone marrow infiltration, the risks and the costs of high-dose therapy necessitating autologous transplantation can only be justified if a significant therapeutic advantage results over conventional radiochemotherapy. Reduction of the risk of relapse achieved through the higher antineoplastic efficacy of high-dose therapy has further to be weighed against its nonhematopoietic toxicities.

The need to retransfuse cryopreserved hematopoietic stem cells after TBI-containing protocols has unequivocally been demonstrated in the allogeneic or syngeneic transplantation settings. For the vast majority of high-dose chemotherapy protocols used with autologous stem cell support, however, only very few comparative studies have been performed with the aim to demonstrate the therapeutic benefit of stem cell retransfusion in shortening the period of myelosuppression or pancytopenia. Due to the substantial bone marrow toxicity associated with most of the current high-dose protocols, it appears reasonable to assume that autologous stem cell support represents an effective supportive therapeutic measure. It should always be kept in mind, however, that the sequelae of previous cytotoxic therapies and, in particular, the aplasiogenic remission-induction protocols currently used in the treatment of acute leukemias can lead to a substantial reduction in the number and proliferative capacity of hematopoietic stem cells. In addition, damage to the cells of the bone marrow microenvironment, which can be also crucial for the reconstitution of the retransfused stem cells, has to be considered.

In principle, autologous stem cell transplantation has certain advantages compared with allogeneic transplantation:

1. It is more widely applicable, because the identification of a histocompatible marrow donor, which largely restricts the use of allogeneic transplantation, is not required.
2. It is not accompanied by immunological complications, like graft rejection or GvHD. This results in a substantially lower therapy-related morbidity and mortality as well as in lower costs of autologous stem cell support.
3. It is better tolerated by elderly patients.

These advantages have to be weighed against the disadvantages of autologous stem cell sources. A putative immunologic antitumor effect, circumstantially evident after allogeneic BMT, is missing after autologous stem cell support. Particularly in leukemic diseases, in lymphatic neoplasias, and in some solid tumors there is further a potential risk to reinoculate clonogenic tumor cells with the graft.

Numerous working groups are endeavored to solve the problem of an occult contamination of the graft through techniques that selectively eliminate tumor cells, which is also referred to as tumor cell purging. The theoretical basis for this approach is that these separation techniques can distinguish between neoplastic cells and hematopoietic stem cells through differing antigen structures on the cell surface membranes or through differing sensitivities to cytotoxic pharmacological treatment. In nonhematologic neoplasias, monoclonal antibodies which are targeted to antigens preferably expressed on the malignant cells are used to achieve a selective reduction of neoplastic cells. Similarly, lymphatic neoplastic cells can be distinguished by a predominance of differentiation antigens, and monoclonal antibodies directed to these antigens are able to eliminate most of the neoplastic population. In acute myeloid leukemia (AML), on the other hand, there is nearly complete phenotypic conformity between clonogenic leukemic and physiologic progenitor cells, which makes selective elimination using monoclonal antibodies directed to differentiation antigens not suitable. Alternatively, in vitro incubation with cytotoxic agents is being attempted in AML. Only the in vitro active oxazaphosphorine derivatives 4-hydroperoxycyclophosphamide and mafosfamide have appreciably been tested in uncontrolled clinical BMT trials. Retrospective analyses performed by the EBMTG, using compiled transplant results from European centers on AML patients, suggest that bone marrow transplants purged by mafosfamide have a positive influence on the risk of relapse and disease-free survival as compared to marrow grafts treated by other purging techniques, or unmanipulated marrow. The limited patient numbers in distinct prognostic patient groups, undefined patient selection criteria and nonstandardized purging and transplant procedures between centers, however, currently preclude definitive conclusions regarding the usefulness of mafosfamide purging in AML. In general, the therapeutic benefit of all the different approaches to tumor cell depletion from autologous stem cell grafts needs to be proven by appropriate prospective comparative trials, and a number of clinical trials in different hematologic and solid-tumor entities are currently performed to investigate this issue. In considering the frequency of relapses in patients with acute leukemias after syngeneic transplantation as a model for the transplantation of tumor cell-free "autologous" marrow, it appears evident that the problem of leukemic relapse after autologous transplantation is predominately caused by the insufficient antileukemic efficacy of current high-dose therapeutic regimens.

During recent years the field of autotransplantation has dramatically changed by the development of methods for harvesting hematopoietic progenitor cells, not from the bone marrow cavities but from the patient's peripheral blood. After the recognition that increased frequencies of hematopoietic progenitor cells are detectable in the peripheral blood of patients recovering from chemotherapy, techniques for the mobilization and harvesting of peripheral blood progenitor cells (PBPC) have rapidly advanced, and autologous PBPC transfusions are now broadly applicable as supportive therapy of high-dose radiochemotherapy. These developments were influenced to a large extent by the availability of recombinant hematopoietic growth factors, especially granulocyte-colony-stimulating factor (G-CSF). This growth factor, among others, has proven efficacy in mobilizing sufficient amounts of PBPC alone or in combination with conventional chemotherapy, which allow accelerated neutrophil and platelet reconstitution after myelosuppressive radiochemotherapy. Besides improvements in leukapheresis techniques for PBPC harvesting, the reliable and rapid quantification of PBPC by the flow-cytometric identification of the CD34 cell surface membrane antigen as their phenotypic surrogate marker represents an important diagnostic advance for the clinical application of autologous PBPC transplantation. The cell population expressing the CD34 antigen in PBPC preparations, however, is clearly heterogeneous and contains a high proportion of committed hematopoietic progenitor cells. One important objection against the application of autologous PBPC after irreversible myeloablative therapy therefore remains the currently unresolved question whether mobilized PBPC preparations contain sufficient amounts of pluripotent hematopoietic stem cells which guarantee permanent hematopoietic reconstitution. Although most of the currently investigated high-dose chemotherapy protocols are very myelosuppressive, they do not lead to eradication of the pluripotent hematopoietic stem cell compartment. Only very few studies have so far investigated myeloablative regimens, like TBI-containing regimens, with autologous PBPC transplantation, and it remains to be seen whether this approach will lead to durable and complete hematopoietic reconstitution.

Whether PBPC preparations have advantages over bone marrow autotransplants with regard to tumor cell contamination has so far not sufficiently been studied in the majority of tumor entities. There is growing evidence, however, that certain techniques for PBPC mobilization can also mobilize tumor cells into the peripheral blood. The currently available data on this issue indicate that, in patients with advanced disease stages, tumor cell contamination apparently presents a similar problem in the different stem cell sources.

A further rapidly evolving field in autologous stem cell support is the positive selection of CD34 antigen-positive cells by immunoadsorption columns or by immunomagnetic separation techniques. These techniques provide the opportunity to purify and enrich hematopoietic progenitor cells, which, at the same time, results in a depletion of contaminating cells. Thus, these positive selection techniques have the potential to be used as a tool for reducing contaminating malignant cells in the graft and for extracting hematopoietic progenitor populations which then may also be further processed ex vivo.

Again, it remains to be proven whether a reduced tumor cell contamination in positively selected CD34 antigen-positive cell preparations will be associated with a decreased risk of disease recurrence after high-dose therapy supported by autotransplantation. Even if these techniques were able to remove all contaminating tumor cells from an autograft, it can be expected that the influence on relapse rates will, at best, be modest because of the high background relapse rates resulting from residual tumor cells surviving high-dose therapy. Nevertheless, the clinical application of tumor cell purging appears justified as long as the advantageous properties of PBPC autotransplants, like the acceleration of neutrophil and platelet reconstitution, are not offset by these techniques.

Important future developments in autotransplantation, which are close to clinical application, include mobilization protocols using combinations of growth factors, the selective expansion of hematopoietic progenitors ex vivo, and somatic gene transfer into hematopoietic cells for the treatment of inherited genetic diseases and for tumor therapy.

12.1. Techniques of Autologous Transplantation

The technique of marrow harvest is identical to that described for allogeneic BMT. Based on data from animal experiments, the minimum efficient cell dose needed for hematopoietic reconstitution after autologous transplantation is reduced by one log as compared to allogeneic transplantation. Enumeration of the growth of colony-forming hematopoietic progenitors in semisolid media from a marrow or PBPC sample is generally used as a semiquantitative in vitro culture assay for the evaluation of the graft progenitor cell content. Most of these assays (CFU-GM, CFU-GEMM, BFU-E) measure committed and mature progenitors. Therefore, these assays are only useful as indicators for the early hematopoietic reconstitution, while more primitive stem cells providing long-term reconstitution cannot be detected with these culture techniques. Major disadvantages of these functional progenitor culture assays include variations between laboratories, lack of standardization, relatively high costs, and low performance. During recent years it became evident that the quantification of CD34 antigen-positive hematopoietic progenitor cells may be useful as a rapid and reliable marker for the progenitor cell content of marrow or PBPC preparations. The available data indicate that the quantification of CD34-positive cells shows a good correlation with CFU-GM measurements and with the kinetics of neutrophil and platelet reconstitution after high-dose myelosuppressive therapy. In addition, peripheral blood CD34-positive cell measurements are now generally used to predict the best time point at which leukapheresis for PBPC harvesting should be performed. It has been estimated that $2.0–5.0 \times 10^6$ CD34-positive cells per kg of body weight are required to attain rapid neutrophil and platelet reconstitution after autologous PBPC transplantation. However, it appears necessary to further define these threshold cell dosages because they may vary with certain characteristics of the procedure, such as the type of mobilization technique or high-dose preparative regimen used, or the application of posttransplant hematopoietic growth factors.

The use of autologous transplantation requires effective cryopreservation of hematopoietic stem cells to bridge the time period in which the high-dose therapy is performed. Despite the limitations of hematopoietic progenitor cell assays, an estimation of the proliferative capacity of the patient's marrow with these assays should be a mandatory component of the pretransplant examinations. In addition, determining the total number of progenitor cells before freezing and after thawing can serve as a control for the quality of cryopreservation. Important aspects to be observed during freezing, storage and thawing of marrow cell suspensions are summarized in table 16. As an intracellular cryoprotective agent, 10% dimethylsulfoxide (DMSO) is generally used. Since, in contrast to marrow cells, granulocytes cannot be cryopreserved by DMSO, contamination of the marrow cell suspension with granulocytes results in lysis of these cells during thawing. This, in turn, leads to release of nucleoproteins and lysosomal enzymes which may cause cell clumping and jelly formation. To avoid this problem, the marrow cell suspension is generally concentrated by cell separation techniques, which allow enrichment of progenitor cells and largely eliminate granulocytes. For the freezing of marrow cells, automatic freezers with defined programmable cooling rates are now generally in use. A particularly critical point in the freezing process is the phase in which the heat of crystallization is released (transition phase) (fig. 17), since warming can lead to a loss of cell viability due to mechanical or toxic damage. By increasing the freezing rate at the beginning of the transition phase ("overcooling"), a temperature increase can be avoided and the transition phase can be kept short. Deep-frozen grafts are stored in liquid nitrogen at a constant temperature of –196 °C. The thawing process must be kept short in order to prevent recrystallization. This can be achieved by putting the freezing bag in a water bath of 40 °C. Although in most instances, DMSO can be infused with relatively few adverse effects after appropriate premedication, washing out the substance in a series of dilution steps gives a greater osmotic stability to the cell suspension, and prevents or diminishes any direct cytotoxic effects of DMSO. The cryopreservation of PBPC is basically identical with the procedure of marrow cells. Although the cell concentrations are usually up to 10-fold higher in preparations of PBPC compared to marrow, this seems to have no negative impact on the quality of progenitor cell viability after cryopreservation.

Table 16. Effective cryopreservation of human bone marrow cells

The Freezing Process
Cell concentration 20–40 × 10^6/ml
Cryoprotective agent (e.g. DMSO)
Constant, slow cooling rate (1–3 °C/min) before and after the transition phase
Freezing bags of polyolefin or teflon-capton
Compression of bags between aluminium plates to ensure homogeneous freezing
Storage
At lowest constant temperature (-196 °C) with constant temperature control to detect any accidental warming
Thawing
Very fast thawing to avoid recrystallization
Stepwise dilution of the cell suspension
Alternative with high cell counts, direct infusion of the cell suspension (within 15 min) via a central venous catheter

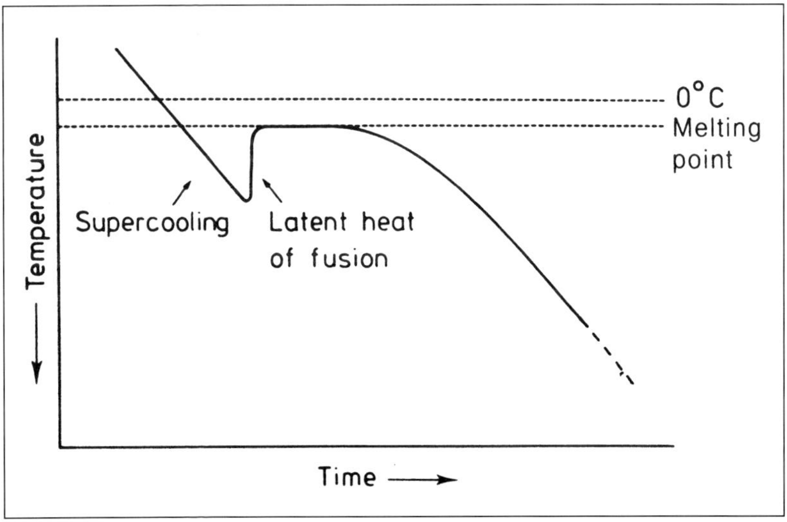

Fig. 17. Schematic temperature – time curve during cryopreservation of bone marrow cells.

12.2. Indications for High-Dose Therapy Followed by Autologous Transplantation

12.2.1. Acute Myeloid Leukemia

High-dose radiochemotherapy followed by retransfusion of autologous bone marrow cells harvested and cryopreserved during remission is presently being investigated in uncontrolled and prospective controlled clinical studies as a consolidation therapy in patients with AML in first or second CR who lack a suitable bone marrow donor. Most of the prospective randomized studies investigating the value of autologous BMT in first CR compared with conventional remission-maintaining chemotherapeutic approaches have failed to demonstrate a higher antileukemic efficacy of high-dose therapy followed by autologous marrow support. A matched-pair analysis performed by the German Cooperative AML Study on Consolidation by Autologous BMT compared with a monthly cyclic maintenance chemotherapy performed over a time period of 3 years showed comparable rates of continuous remissions and no significant differences in disease-free survival or in overall survival. However, in the light of the comparable antileukemic efficacy and therapy-related risks, one important argument in favor of autologous BMT might be that patients would be spared the burden of prolonged chemotherapy. An ongoing prospective randomized MRC trial suggests that the risk of recurrence is significantly reduced by 20% after high-dose therapy and autologous BMT performed during first CR compared to consolidation therapy alone. Despite the lowered risk of a relapse in this study, there is still no survival advantage for patients after autologous BMT.

A retrospective analysis by the EBMTG suggested that the treatment results of autologous BMT during first CR are significantly influenced by the time interval between achievement of remission and high-dose therapy. The relapse rates ranged from around 65%, if therapy was performed within 3 months after entering remission, to around 35%, if remission duration was longer than 6 months. These differences can most probably be explained by a patient selection bias, because patients with very short remission durations have a lower chance to undergo autologous BMT. Therefore, autologous transplant results obtained in patients with prolonged remission duration are positively biased by the exclusion of early relapses.

To what extent an ex vivo treatment of autologous marrow cells aimed at reducing the content of clonogenic leukemic cells by incubation with activated cyclophosphamide derivatives or by monoclonal antibodies influences the relapse incidence is currently judged controversial. In the above mentioned retrospective analysis, patients who received bone marrow treated ex vivo attained a marginal advantage with regard to disease-free survival, if they were treated within 6 months after achieving CR and TBI was part of the high-dose therapy preceding autologous marrow support. The fact that relapses might not exclusively be caused by residual leukemic cells that survive high-dose radiochemotherapy, but may also result from the retransfusion of leukemic cells along with the autologous graft has been illuminated by studies, in which bone marrow cells labeled with the neomycin-resistant gene were retransfused. These genetic markers could subsequently be retraced during relapse. Future studies on patients with disease-specific genetic markers will contribute to elucidating the relative significance between residual leukemic cells in the patient or in the graft and the development of leukemic relapse after autologous transplantations.

Uncontrolled studies describe rates of continuous remissions of up to 25% in advanced stages of AML after high-dose therapy and autologous BMT. Hence, autologous BMT represents a therapeutic option in patients without histocompatible donors after the first relapse if a graft obtained during the first or second CR is available.

More recent approaches are testing the value of immunomodulating methods, e.g., with cyclic interleukin-2 administration after high-dose therapy supported by autologous BMT to induce an additional antileukemic effect.

12.2.2. Acute Lymphoblastic Leukemia

The value of autologous BMT in the treatment concept of ALL has not yet been clearly established by any of the published studies investigating this issue. In patients without an HLA-identical bone marrow donor, the indications for high-dose therapy followed by autologous blood or marrow stem cell support are being tested, analogously to the indications for allogeneic BMT, predominantly in second CR as part of the German Cooperative ALL clinical studies in adults and children. In patients whose disease is characterized by factors indicating an increased risk of relapse, high-dose therapy with stem cell support is presently being examined even in first CR, if an HLA-identical related or unrelated marrow donor has not been identified.

In contrast to AML, techniques for selective ex vivo depletion of residual leukemic cells from the bone marrow are available by using differentiation-specific monoclonal antibodies. The effectiveness of bone marrow immunopurging can subsequently be tested by amplification of leukemia clone-specific DNA or RNA. As already outlined for AML, such studies will contribute to illuminating the importance of minimal leukemic cell contamination in the transplant not detectable by conventional diagnostic techniques with regard to the risk of relapse. One clinical study, using molecular genetic analysis for the detection of minimal residual disease in patients with low-grade malignant lymphoma, suggests that the ex vivo depletion of bcl2-oncogene-positive lymphoma cells below the sensitivity threshold of molecular genetic detection might improve disease-free survival after autologous BMT.

The question is completely open as to whether high-dose therapy with subsequent transfusion of peripheral blood stem cells poses an alternative to autologous BMT in high-risk ALL patients. The potential contamination of peripheral blood stem cell preparations with clonogenic leukemia cells might be counteracted by using techniques for the positive enrichment of pluripotent progenitor cells of hematopoiesis which express no lymphatic differentiation antigens.

12.2.3. Chronic Myeloid Leukemia

Various approaches for autologous BMT or peripheral stem cell transplantation are currently being investigated in patients without suitable marrow donors. In the past it was shown that patients in advanced stages of CML achieved at least a short second chronic phase induced by high-dose radiochemotherapy followed by the transfusion of bone marrow or blood stem cells which had been harvested and cryopreserved during the second chronic phase. More recent concepts attempt to augment the growth of residual normal hematopoiesis in vivo by high-dose chemotherapy or IFN-α therapy in order to obtain stem cells with a reduced content of Ph'-positive cells from the bone marrow or peripheral blood. In vitro approaches with various modifications of long-term bone marrow culture techniques exploit the distinct proliferative behavior of normal and leukemic hematopoiesis in order to selectively augment normal hematopoiesis. Proof has meanwhile been obtained that cytogenetically normal precursor cells can be obtained in vitro from patients in the chronic phase and be expanded. After high-dose radiochemotherapy and transferal of these cells, isolated cases of long-term complete or partial cytogenetic remissions were reported. Maintenance therapy with IFN-α after BMT or peripheral stem cell transplantation is also a subject of current investigations. It is presently not possible to estimate the curative potential of these various approaches. The transplantation results with bone marrow of identical twin donors achieved in CML during the chronic phase hold the promise that at best 50% of the patients will sustain a disease-free status due to the insufficient antileukemic efficacy of radiochemotherapy and to the lack of a GvL effect.

12.2.4. Non-Hodgkin's Lymphoma

12.2.4.1. Intermediate- and High-Grade Malignant Lymphomas

At diagnosis, the majority of patients with intermediate- or high-grade malignant non-Hodgkin's lymphomas are in a stage of dissemination which extends beyond localized lymph node involvement. Polychemotherapeutic regimens including anthracyclines in combination with local radiotherapy of the primary tumor site can achieve CR in 50–60% of patients in nonlocalized stages of the disease. However, lymphoma recurs in approximately half of these patients. Despite some improvements in the therapeutic outcome after disease recurrence, definitive cures are the exception in this situation. The following prognostic factors at the time of diagnosis were identified in metaanalyses conducted in large-scale clinical studies (favorable vs. unfavorable): patient age (< 60 years vs. ≥ 60 years), performance status (ECOG grade < 2 vs. ≥ 2), dissemination stage (< III vs. ≥ III), extranodal involvement (no extranodal involvement vs. extranodal involvement), and LDH serum activity (normal vs. elevated).

Similar to leukemic diseases, high-grade non-Hodgkin's lymphomas frequently are characterized by a steep slope of the cytotoxic dose-response relationship curve. Consequently, the concept of high-dose therapy supported by hematopoietic stem cells is also increasingly used in these disease entities.

Based on current experience it can be concluded that the major influential factors predictive for the successful application of high-dose therapy in this heterogeneous group of diseases comprise disease stage, extent of previous exposure to cytotoxic therapy, response (sensitive relapse) or nonresponse (refractory relapse) to conventional chemotherapy given during disease recurrence, the presence of concurrent diseases as well as the performance status of the afflicted patients. If there has been no response to conventional chemotherapy and the patient's performance status is very poor, the incidence of therapy-related complications and tumor recurrence rates are so unacceptably high that common opinion has meanwhile rejected high-dose therapy as an "ultima ratio" in therapy-refractory end stages of non-Hodgkin's lymphomas. A growing number of clinical trials now include high-dose therapeutic regimens in the overall treatment concepts of malignant lymphomas, preferably as high-dose consolidation treatment of first CR or as a salvage treatment after the first chemosensitive relapse.

Most previously published studies on high-dose therapy in patients with malignant lymphomas were conducted in conjunction with the retransfusion of autologous bone marrow stem cells. Now that it has been shown that hematopoietic regeneration takes a more rapid course after transfusion of peripheral blood stem cells as compared to bone marrow stem cells, it can be expected that future clinical studies will primarily use autologous blood stem cells to support high-dose therapy. Recently, studies on the combined use of bone marrow and blood stem cells have also been reported. It still remains to be seen, however, whether the accelerated hematopoietic regeneration connected with the peripheral blood stem cell support can favorably influence the clinical results of high-dose therapy. The accelerated hematopoietic regeneration obtained by peripheral blood stem cell support will allow repeated applications of high-dose therapy in the future, which may result in an enhancement of the therapeutic intensity and, in consequence, of the curative potential.

Allogeneic BMT plays a subordinate role in patients with high-grade malignant non-Hodgkin's lymphoma. As anticipated, it has been demonstrated that the therapy-related mortality is higher and relapse rates tend to be lower after allogeneic BMT than after autologous BMT, without any distinct advantage with regard to disease-free survival being currently recognizable for either of these techniques. A hypothetical advantage favoring allogeneic BMT might consist of an immunological antitumor effect of the allogeneic graft in terms of a "graft-versus-lymphoma" effect, similar to that circumstantially observed in leukemic diseases. If a suitable donor is available within the family, disseminated lymphoma infiltrations of the bone marrow or a very high risk of relapse might be arguments which speak for the application of an allogeneic transplant in exceptional cases. In the same sense, future studies must investigate the indication for BMT with histocompatible unrelated bone marrow donors in patients with prognostically unfavorable lymphoma entities.

As already mentioned, the morbidity and mortality of high-dose therapeutic regimens are primarily dependent on the disease stage and on the patient's performance status. In first or second CR of intermediate or high-grade malignant lymphomas, the rate of fatal complications after autologous stem cell transplantations is less than 10%, increasing to 20% after allogeneic BMT. In advanced disease stages, the therapy-related mortality is particularly higher due to fatal infectious complications. If mediastinal irradiation has been performed as a part of the primary treatment, the frequency of fatal interstitial pneumonias increases markedly as a result of the cumulative pulmonary toxicity.

At present, predominantly chemotherapeutic high-dose regimens are applied in malignant lymphomas. Commonly used combinations consist of the cytotoxic drugs cyclophosphamide, BCNU and etoposide (CVB regimen), BCNU, etoposide, cytosine arabinoside and melphalan (BEAM regimen), or busulfan and cyclophosphamide (BUCY regimen). To date, none of the aforementioned, or other, high-dose therapeutic regimens have demonstrated a clear therapeutic advantage. Aiming to further enhance the tumoricidal effect, dose escalation studies of single or multiple components of the above regimens are currently ongoing. In the light of mortality rates of around 10% associated with the use of the above high-dose regimens, it can be expected that intensification of therapy solely by escalating the dose of cytotoxic drugs will not contribute to improving disease-free survival.

One aspect receiving increasing attention in high-dose therapy of malignant lymphomas is the inclusion of adjuvant involved-field irradiation of the sites of relapse or the initial main tumor bulk. Adjuvant radiotherapy should be limited to a maximum target volume dose of 28 Gy, if irradiation is given in the immediate time frame of high-dose therapy. According to current experience, adjuvant irradiation lowers the probability of local lymphoma relapses without increasing the rate of treatment-related complications.

Based on a retrospective multicenter analysis published in 1987, which included patients with heterogeneous histological subtypes and disease stages of intermediate- and high-grade lymphomas, response to preceding conventional therapy and the disease stage at the time of high-dose therapy were the most important prognostic factors affecting disease-free survival after high-dose therapy. The overwhelming prognostic significance of these two factors has meanwhile been confirmed by a number of studies.

Various approaches to the ex vivo purging of residual lymphoma cells from the bone marrow by means of differentiation-specific monoclonal antibodies or chemotherapeutic agents have not yet yielded consistent results with regard to the question of whether the relapse risk can be substantially reduced by purging techniques. The results of clinical studies applying these approaches remain difficult to interpret because of the methodologic problems in demonstrating purging efficacy. The growing availability of sensitive molecular genetic methods for the demonstration of minimal residual disease in lymphoma patients should hold the future promise of contributing to clarify the efficacy of these approaches. Therefore, future clinical studies must also elucidate how occult contamination of stem cell preparations with residual lymphoma cells affects the risk of recurrence by using disease-specific molecular genetic markers, like the bcl2 oncogene, as an integral part of the clinical monitoring. Presently, the question still remains open as to whether and under which conditions qualitative and/or quantitative differences exist in the lymphoma cell contamination of stem cell preparations obtained from the peripheral blood or bone marrow.

Over 70% of lymphoma relapses after high-dose therapy manifest in the regions of earlier involvement. The majority of recurrences develops within the 1st year, and only in exceptional cases later than 3 years after high-dose therapy. Involvement of the bone marrow at the time of diagnosis or during relapse had no adverse effect on disease-free survival after high-dose therapy with autologous bone marrow stem cell substitution in patients with both Hodgkin's and non-Hodgkin's lymphomas. These observations might be interpreted to imply that, similar to the situation in acute leukemias, retransfused occult lymphoma cells have no relevant impact on the development of relapses. The fact that lymphoma recurrences predominantly occur in regions of previous involvement suggests that the tumoricidal potential of high-dose therapy in these regions was not sufficient. It appears rather unlikely, on the other hand, that local factors could promote the growth of retransfused lymphoma cells in previously affected regions.

Another controversial aspect is the administration of hematopoietic growth factors after high-dose therapy supported by hematopoietic stem cells. Although it has been unequivocally demonstrated that the prophylactic use of granulocyte-colony-stimulating factor (G-CSF) or granulocyte-macrophage-colony-stimulating factor (GM-CSF) shortens the duration of the critical granulocytopenia after high-dose therapy (as after dose-escalated conventional chemotherapy), the effect of the prophylactic administration of these hematopoietins on relevant clinical end points like frequency of infections, duration of systemic antibiotic therapy or the number of febrile days was not as convincing as initially expected. After weighing the clinical benefit against the high expenses connected with the prophylactic use of hematopoietic growth factors as part of the high-dose therapy of lymphatic neoplasms, their application can be recommended only if the critical granulocytopenia concentration of $< 0.5 \times 10^9$/l is expected to last at least 7 days.

Table 17 presents an outline of the recommendations of an International Consensus Conference (June 4-6, 1993 in Lyon) made with regard to the administration of high-dose therapy supported by hematopoietic stem cells in malignant lymphomas. Especially in Anglo-Saxon countries, in France and in Italy, the number of patients treated with high-dose therapy has increased dramatically within the past years. Against the backdrop of this development, a critical note should be made that the superior efficacy of high-dose therapy compared to conventional radiochemotherapy in malignant lymphomas has so far been proven only by a single prospective randomized study (PARMA study) in patients with chemotherapy-sensitive relapses of intermediate or high-grade malignant non-Hodgkin's lymphoma. This cooperative study demonstrated that patients randomized to the high-dose therapy arm had a significant reduction in the risk of relapse and a significant survival advantage .

The preponderant number of published clinical studies on high-dose therapy in malignant lymphoma bases the assessment of its value on comparisons with historical data of conventional radiochemotherapy. Although such studies are indispensable for developing study designs, they do not provide a reliable judgement as to whether high-dose therapy regimens are actually superior to conventional therapy modalities. They involve too many difficult-to-evaluate factors, such as non-uniform patient selection criteria, heterogeneous diseases and stages, different types of pretreatment and supportive therapy, etc. A prospective randomized study conducted in Belgium and France on a total of 370 patients with high-grade malignant non-Hodgkin's lymphoma (LNH-87) has yet to prove any significant survival benefit for patients who had been treated with high-dose therapy as part of the primary treatment. Several randomized studies had to be terminated because the treating physicians and the afflicted patients judged the high-dose therapy to be the more effective option and were therefore frequently not in agreement with the idea of randomization.

In conclusion, it can be stated on the basis of previously published results that high-dose therapy supported by hematopoietic stem cells can achieve sustained re-

Table 17. Recommendations of the Consensus Conference (Lyon, France, June 1993) on intensive chemotherapy plus hematopoietic stem cell transplantation in adult patients with malignant lymphomas

	Primary therapy	Relapse	Primary-resistant
Intermediate- or high-grade non-Hodgkin's lymphomas	conventional chemotherapy vs. high-dose therapy in patients with a high risk of relapse	complete PARMA study or initiate similiar studies	phase I/II studies
Low-grade non-Hodgkin's lymphomas	no consensus	phase III studies: conventional chemotherapy vs. high-dose therapy	phase III studies: conventional chemotherapy vs. high-dose therapy
Advanced Hodgkin's lymphomas	await better prognostic factors for the identification of patients with an increased risk of relapse	phase III studies: conventional chemotherapy vs. high dose therapy	phase I/II studies

missions in 40–50% of patients with recurrent intermediate- and high-grade malignant non-Hodgkin's lymphomas. Although the results of high-dose therapy in the primary treatment and in early stages of these lymphoma entities hold future promise, they must be subjected to further validation in prospective randomized comparisons with conventional radiochemotherapy taking into account well-defined prognostic factors. Conversely, studies comparing different high-dose therapeutic regimens, varying stem cell sources, the influence of recombinant hematopoietins, and the value of techniques for purging residual lymphoma cells from stem cell preparations are of secondary importance. These topics should not be dealt with until the fundamental questions have been clarified in the framework of clinical studies.

12.2.4.2. Low-Grade Malignant Lymphomas

With the rare exception of strictly localized stages at diagnosis, low-grade malignant lymphomas cannot be curatively treated by current therapeutic modalities. However, many patients do experience a stable course of their disease over years, requiring only minor therapeutic interventions and barely restricting the patient's quality of life (indolent disease). This has also been observed in patients in disseminated stages. In up to 20% of afflicted patients, even intermittent tumor remissions unrelated to therapy have been observed. The significant factors prognostic of survival in untreated patients with disseminated stages of the disease appear to be the calculated total tumor mass and patient sex. In male patients with a high tumor mass (most unfavorable prognostic subgroup), mean survival was around 3.5 years, while 92% of female patients with low tumor mass were still alive after 10 years. Parallel to the situation in multiple myeloma, the serum level of β_2-microglobulin (< 3 or ≥ 3 mg/l) is an important predictor of the attainment of remission.

To date, there has been no reliable evidence indicating that polychemotherapeutic measures can prolong survival in patients with low-grade malignant non-Hodgkin's lymphomas. Therefore, a compelling indication for chemotherapy is given predominantly in case of symptomatic disease progression. This wait-and-see therapeutic attitude particularly applies to lymphocytic lymphoma and its leukemic variant, chronic lymphatic leukemia, to lymphoplasmocytoid immunocytoma and centroblastic-centrocytic lymphoma according to the Kiel classification. Conversely, initial chemotherapy is deemed justified in patients with centrocytic lymphoma, because of their poorer median survival rates. The standard therapy in virtually all forms of low-grade malignant non-Hodgkin's lymphoma is considered to be the combination of cyclophosphamide, vincristine and prednisone (COP regimen), which has proven equipotent, even in comparison with intensified, specifically anthracycline-containing chemotherapeutic regimens. New studies are testing whether IFN-α can increase the rate of polychemotherapy-induced CRs in advanced low-grade malignant non-Hodgkin's lymphomas or prolong the duration of remission. Based on the results of phase II studies with the new purine analogues chlorodeoxyadenosine, deoxycoformycin, and particularly fludarabine, it can be expected that, at least in a proportion of patients with chronic lymphatic leukemia, complete and sustained hematologic remissions can be achieved.

Approaches to high-dose therapy in low-grade malignant non-Hodgkin's lymphoma have just been recently investigated. In one study including 69 patients with recurrent low-grade malignant B-cell lymphomas who achieved a complete or partial remission with conventional chemotherapy and were subsequently treated with high-dose therapy supported by autologous bone marrow stem cells, therapy-associated mortality was 4% and disease-free 2-year survival was 53%. The remission status at the time of high-dose therapy was the most important predictor of disease-free survival, which was 80% for patients in CR as opposed to 20% in patients with partial remission after a follow-up period of 2 years. Despite these promising but preliminary results, it remains to be seen whether high-dose therapy concepts can contribute to an improvement of survival or have curative potential in low-grade malignant non-Hodgkin's lymphoma. As given in table 17, clinical studies should primarily investigate the value of high-dose therapy in advanced or primary refractory stages of low-grade malignant non-Hodgkin's lymphoma in comparison with conventional radiochemotherapy. Several such studies have now been initiated.

12.2.5. Hodgkin's Disease

Especially in early and localized, but even in intermediate and advanced stages of Hodgkin's lymphoma, the curative potential of conventional radio- and chemotherapy is high, compared with the results of therapy in non-Hodgkin's lymphoma. Patients in early stages without risk factors rarely suffer a relapse after adequate local radiotherapy. Even in the case of a relapse, long-term remissions and cures can be achieved in this group of patients by conventional therapeutic modalities, thus reserving the question of high-dose therapy for exceptional cases only. A high percentage of relapsing pediatric patients with primarily advanced stages of Hodgkin's lymphoma can be curatively treated by conventional radiochemotherapy. In contrast, relapsing adults with initially advanced disease stages have a minimal chance of cure with conventional therapy, if relapses occur within the first 12 months after entering remission and B symptoms are present at the time of relapse. The predictive value of the recognized prognostic factors for relapse after successful primary therapy of advanced stages of Hodgkin's lymphoma is presently below 50%. Even in initially advanced disease stages, more than half of the patients remain disease-free. Moreover, patients with a high risk of relapse cannot be identified with a sufficient degree of certainty. Therefore, high-dose therapeutic concepts necessitating hematopoietic stem cell support are not being investigated as part of the first-line therapy of intermediate and advanced Hodgkin's lymphoma, but rather virtually exclusively during relapse. According to currently published results of noncomparative studies, high-dose therapy achieved sustained remissions in 20–60% of patients with intermediate or advanced stages of Hodgkin's lymphoma after first relapse. Metaanalyses of these studies suggest that the response to conventional salvage therapy, the patient's performance status, and a previous bone marrow involvement are decisive for predicting the efficacy of high-dose therapy. Single studies on the use of high-dose therapy with stem cell support as first-line therapy of Hodgkin's lymphomas have also been reported. For the reasons discussed above, this treatment option as part of the first-line therapy appears not justifiable on the basis of adverse prognostic factors.

Following the recommendations of an International Consensus Conference (table 17), the value of high-dose therapy supported by autologous stem cells should primarily be investigated after the first relapse of disease in adult patients with initially advanced Hodgkin's lymphoma in comparison to conventional second-line therapy. This approach is presently being investigated by the German Cooperative Hodgkin's Disease Relapse Study (HD-R1). This prospective randomized study compares a conventional high-dose second-line chemotherapy with high-dose chemotherapy necessitating stem cell support. The German Cooperative Hodgkin's Disease Study (HD-9) further investigates the value of a time-intensified high-dose therapy supported by hematopoietic growth factors (BEACOPP regimen) with the same regimen at basic dosages, and with a standard induction therapy consisting of 3 double cycles COPP-ABVD as the primary treatment of patients with advanced Hodgkin's lymphoma. This study design should also allow future conclusions with regard to the potential value of hematopoietic stem cell-supported high-dose therapy in the primary management of advanced Hodgkin's lymphoma.

12.2.6. Multiple Myeloma

With the exception of strictly localized stages (solitary plasmacytoma), multiple myeloma also presents an entity which cannot be curatively managed by conventional radiochemotherapeutic modalities. More recent studies prove that the assessment of disease dynamics is of great prognostic importance besides the Durie-Salmon staging of tumor burden. This connection was also confirmed by the German Cooperative Myeloma Study which found no tumor progression in about 20% of patients with initial stage II disease over longer observation periods (smoldering myeloma). Thus, patients with spontaneously nonprogressive courses and those with isolated gammopathies of unclear etiology must be distinguished from patients with progressive myeloma. However, classification into various prognostic groups is occasionally only possible by monitoring the course of the disease. Another problem with regard to assessing and comparing therapeutic strategies is the presently nonuniform definition of remission in multiple myeloma.

In multiple myeloma, response to chemotherapeutic measures is not necessarily correlated with survival. Standard therapy is still the cyclic administration of a combination of melphalan and prednisone, and survival rates achieved by this therapy are comparable with the results of more aggressive polychemotherapeutic regimens. The median survival in progressive myeloma is around 3 years. Efforts to improve this poor prognosis with various strategies of maintenance therapy have not yielded any validated success to date. Although prolonged therapy with IFN-α can extend chemotherapy-induced remissions, it appears to have no effect on survival.

Against this backdrop, the concept of high-dose therapy for the treatment of progressive myeloma was initially examined in younger patients using myeloablative radiochemotherapeutic conditioning followed by transplantation of marrow from histocompatible sibling donors. In a first retrospective analysis conducted by the EBMT, which included 90 patients from European transplant centers, the proportion of patients with sustained hematologic remissions was in the range of 40%, and the relapse rate was around 17% after a median follow-up period of 40 months. Prognostic factors for disease-free survival in this analysis were the initial disease stage, the extent of exposure to previous cytotoxic therapy, patient age, and the response to the conditioning regimen. These prognostic factors have recently been confirmed by a more comprehensive EBMT analysis on more than 300 patients.

In elderly patients and in those without histocompatible marrow donors, high-dose therapy with autologous stem cell support is currently being investigated in clinical studies. The serum level of β_2-microglobulin has been identified in this therapeutic approach as an important prognostic factor for survival in hematologic remission. The currently published study results have provided no evidence suggesting that high-dose therapy with autologous stem cell support, even in patients treated in non-refractory stages, might be a curative approach to progressive myeloma.

In younger patients with progressive plasmacytoma who have a histocompatible related or unrelated donor, clinical studies should primarily be aimed at examining the curative potential of allogeneic BMT. It still remains open whether high-dose therapy with autologous stem cell substitution improves the prognosis of progressive plasmacytoma in comparison to conventional palliative therapy. This question is presently the subject of ongoing prospective comparative studies.

12.2.7. Solid Tumors

High-dose therapeutic concepts are currently being investigated to a rapidly increasing extent in patients with solid tumors in disease stages, who cannot be curatively treated with conventional radiochemotherapy, but still respond to these modalities. In the first-line therapy of solid tumors, high-dose therapy with stem cell support is predominantly being investigated as a remission-induction therapy in patients with a small residual tumor mass or as an adjuvant therapy in patients with unfavorable prognostic disease features at diagnosis. Similarly, high-dose therapeutic concepts are being investigated in chemosensitive tumor relapses for the treatment of residual tumor manifestations and as consolidation therapies of second remissions after successful second-line therapy. Meanwhile, extensive experience has been gained in patients with testicular cancer, small-cell lung cancer, breast cancer, childhood neuroblastoma, Ewing's sarcoma and osteosarcoma. Although high-dose therapy cannot be regarded as an established treatment of these tumor entities, there is growing evidence suggesting that this therapeutic concept might offer advantages in certain, but still undefined, prognostic subgroups of patients.

It has now become apparent that in chemosensitive solid tumors the remission rates can be increased by high-dose therapy. The key questions, however, as to whether the greater remission-inducing potential of high-dose therapy also leads to a prolongation of remission duration and to an improvement of survival in comparison to conventional adjuvant or palliative therapeutic concepts still remain to be answered. In light of the considerable toxicities, discomfort to patients, and expenses associated with high-dose regimens necessitating stem cell support, future studies must appropriately examine whether either conventional or dose-escalated radiochemotherapy supported by hematopoietic growth factors may produce comparable results.

13. Outlook

Allogeneic BMT is now accepted worldwide as a treatment modality for numerous life-threatening diseases of the hematopoietic system. High-dose radiochemotherapy followed by autologous hematopoietic stem cell support is currently broadly investigated as a treatment option for hematologic malignancies and solid tumors.

To further improve the clinical application of allogeneic BMT in the future, major advances have to be achieved in several fields. Prophylaxis and therapy of acute and chronic GvHD are certainly still unsatisfactory, and new approaches to the prevention and treatment of GvHD are clearly warranted. New strategies for the prevention and treatment of bacterial, fungal and viral infections in allogeneic BMT recipients have to be further developed to make the procedure safer and more broadly applicable. Another important issue is the clinical evaluation of the benefits of recombinant hematopoietic growth factors and lymphokines in the settings of allogeneic and autologous transplantation. Alternative hematopoietic stem cell sources, like allogeneic peripheral blood or cord blood cells, are increasingly investigated and may compete with marrow transplantation in the future. Together with progress in tissue typing techniques, the limitations of a broader application of allogeneic marrow transplantation to the majority of patients without suitable donors are going to be diminished by the ever increasing number of volunteer-unrelated donors worldwide. Major efforts have to be directed to a reduction of the toxicity of current conditioning protocols and to improvements in their antitumor efficacy. Another important future field is the engineering of hematopoietic stem cell transplants ex vivo, which is increasingly used for selective expansion of hematopoietic cells, for the depletion of tumor cells contaminating autologous transplants, or for gene transfer into hematopoietic cells.

In general, it can be expected that BMT will continue to gain in importance and that the clinical results can be further improved.

Textbooks

Atkinson K (ed): Clinical Bone Marrow Transplantation: A Reference Textbook. Cambridge, Cambridge University Press, 1994.

Deeg HJ, Klingemann HG, Phillips GL: A Guide to Bone Marrow Transplantation. Berlin, Springer, 1988.

Forman SJ, Blume KG, Thomas ED (eds): Bone Marrow Transplantation. Oxford, Blackwell Scientific, 1994.

Abbreviations

ALL	Acute lymphoblastic leukemia
ALS	Antilymphocyte globulin
AML	Acute myeloid leukemia
ATG	Antithymocyte globulin
AUL	Acute undifferentiated leukemia
B-ALL	ALL expressing B-lymphocyte differentiation antigens (Burkitt's type)
BMFT	Bundesministerium für Forschung und Technik (Ministery for Research and Technology of the Federal Republic of Germany)
CML	Chronic myeloid leukemia
CMV	Cytomegalovirus
CR	Complete remission
DFS	Disease-free survival
EBMT	European Cooperative Group for Bone Marrow Transplantation
FAB	French-American-British
FUO	Fever of unknown origin
GvHD	Graft-versus-host disease
GvHR	Graft-versus-host reaction
GvLR	Graft-versus-leukemia reaction
HLA	Human leukocyte antigen system A
HSV	Herpes simplex virus
HvGR	Host-versus-graft reaction
IBMTR	International Bone Marrow Transplant Registry
IP	Interstitial pneumonia
MHC	Major histocompatibility complex
MLC	Mixed lymphocyte culture
NK	Natural killer cells
PBPC	Peripheral blood progenitor cells
SAA	Severe aplastic anemia
SCID	Severe combined immune deficiency
VOD	Hepatic veno-occlusive disease
VZV	Varicella-zoster virus